AF477170

BIOINFORMATICS:
A PRACTICAL MANUAL

BIOINFORMATICS:
A PRACTICAL MANUAL

Dr. K. Kasturi

and

K. Sri Lakshmi

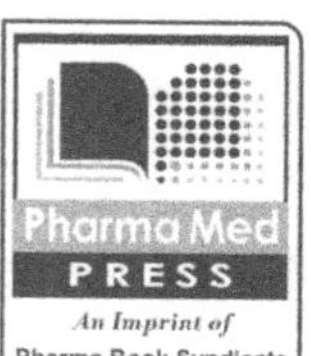

PharmaMed Press

An imprint of Pharma Book Syndicate

4-4-316, Giriraj Lane,
Sultan Bazar, Hyderabad - 500 095.

Published by

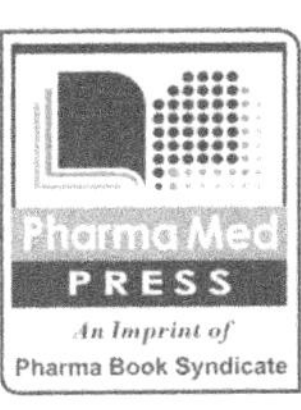

PharmaMed Press

An imprint of Pharma Book Syndicate

4-4-316, Giriraj Lane, Sultan Bazar, Hyderabad - 500 095.

Phone: 040-23445605, 23445688; Fax: 91+40-23445611

E-mail: info@pharmamedpress.com

www.pharmamedpress.com/pharmamedpress.net

ISBN : 978-93-89974-59-1

Preface

The Science of Bioinformatics is important for the professionals in the fields of Biotechnology, Biochemistry and Computer Science.

The Basic practical knowledge about various databases and tools of Bioinformatics have been covered. This provides a perfect practical exposure for students pursuing Bioinformatics at graduate and postgraduate levels. We are greatful to our parents and mentors who have patronized us to fulfil this job. We are especially thankful to the publishers for the service rendered.

- Authors

Contents

1

Biological Databases

A database is a collection of <u>information</u> that is organized so that it can easily be accessed, managed, and updated. In one view, databases can be classified according to types of content: bibliographic, full-text, numeric, and images.

If the information is about Biological Data, such as Nucleotide or Protein sequence, it's secondary or 3D-structure, metabolic pathways, micro-array data and scientific publications etc., then the data base is called Biological Databases.

A primary Biological Databases give information about sequence or structure information alone.

Primary Nucleotide Sequence Database: GenBank, EMBL, DDBJ

Primary Protein Sequence Database: PIR_PSD, Swiss-Prot, TrEMBL,

Primary Structure Database: PDB

A Derived or secondary Database derives the information from primary databases and analyses secondary structure information like signature sequences, motifs, pattern or regular expression, and finger prints etc.

Protein secondary sequence Databases (The derived Databases): Prosite, PRODOM, Pfam, PRINTS etc.

In case of Secondary Structure Databases gives information on classification of proteins based on their structures.

Secondary Structure Databases: CATH, SCOP, DSSP, FSSP, DALI.

The current book describes how to access major databases like

Nucleotide Sequence Database: GenBank

Protein sequence Database: Swissprot

Structure Database: PDB

Note: For nucleic acid sequence databases derived database information is futile unlike proteins, they don't have higher level of organization of structures (primary, secondary, and tertiary, quaternary) as well the DNA structure is constant for almost for all organisms, whereas the proteins differ.

GenBank – The Nucleotide Sequence Database

GenBank® is the NIH genetic sequence database, an annotated collection of all publicly available DNA sequences (*Nucleic Acids Research*, 2008 Jan;36(Database issue):D25-30). There are approximately 85,759,586,764 bases in 82,853,685 sequence records in the traditional GenBank divisions and 108,635,736,141 bases in 27,439,206 sequence records in the WGS division as of February 2008.

The complete release notes for the current version of GenBank are available on the NCBI ftp site. A new release is made every two months. GenBank is part of the International Nucleotide Sequence Database Collaboration, which comprises the DNA DataBank of Japan (DDBJ), the European Molecular Biology Laboratory (EMBL), and GenBank at NCBI. These three organizations exchange data on a daily basis.

GenBank vs. RefSeq

Sequence records are created by scientists who submit sequence data to GenBank. As an archival database, GenBank may contain hundreds of records for the same gene. In addition, because there is no independent review system, the types of information may vary from record to record, and GenBank sequence data may contain errors and contaminant vector DNA. To address some of the problems associated with GenBank sequence records, NCBI developed its RefSeq database.

RefSeq is NCBI's database of reference sequences. RefSeq serves as a curated, non-redundant source of sequence information for genomic DNA contigs (genomic segments constructed by ordering cloned DNA fragments), mRNA transcripts, and proteins associated with known genes. RefSeq records are created and updated as needed by NCBI staff. Since RefSeq records undergo a review process that screens for problems such as sequencing errors and vector contamination, RefSeq records are good sources of sequence information.

RefSeq accession numbers can be distinguished from GenBank accessions by their distinct prefix format of 2 characters followed by an underscore character ('_'). For example, a RefSeq protein accession is NP_015325.

Accession	Molecule	Method @	Note
AC_123456	Genomic	Mixed	Alternate complete genomic molecule. This prefix is used for records that are provided to reflect an alternate assembly or annotation. Primarily used for viral, prokaryotic records.
AP_123456	Protein	Mixed	Protein products; alternate protein record. This prefix is used for records that are provided to reflect an alternate assembly or annotation. The AP_ prefix was originally designated for bacterial proteins but this usage was changed.
NC_123456	Genomic	Mixed	Complete genomic molecules including genomes, chromosomes, organelles, plasmids.
NG_123456	Genomic	Mixed	Incomplete genomic region; supplied to support the NCBI genome annotation pipeline. Represents either non-transcribed pseudogenes, or larger regions representing a gene cluster that is difficult to annotate via automatic methods.
NM_123456 NM_123456789	mRNA	Mixed	Transcript products; mature messenger RNA (mRNA) transcripts.
NP_123456 NP_123456789	Protein	Mixed	Protein products; primarily full-length precursor products but may include some partial proteins and mature peptide products.
NR_123456	RNA	Mixed	Non-coding transcripts including structural RNAs, transcribed pseudogenes, and others.

Contd....

NT_123456	Genomic	Automated	Intermediate genomic assemblies of BAC and/or Whole Genome Shotgun sequence data.
NW_123456 NW_123456789	Genomic	Automated	Intermediate genomic assemblies of BAC or Whole Genome Shotgun sequence data.
NZ_ABCD12345678	Genomic	Automated	A collection of whole genome shotgun sequence data for a project. Accessions are not tracked between releases. The first four characters following the underscore (e.g. 'ABCD') identifies a genome project.
XM_123456 XM_123456789	mRNA	Automated	Transcript products; model mRNA provided by a genome annotation process; sequence corresponds to the genomic contig.
XP_123456 XP_123456789	Protein	Automated	Protein products; model proteins provided by a genome annotation process; sequence corresponds to the genomic contig.
XR_123456	RNA	Automated	Transcript products; model non-coding transcripts provided by a genome annotation process; sequence corresponds to the genomic contig.
YP_123456 YP_123456789	Protein	Mixed	Protein products; no corresponding transcript record provided. Primarily used for bacterial, viral, and mitochondrial records.
ZP_12345678	Protein	Automated	Protein products; annotated on NZ_ accessions (often via computational methods).

Contd....

NS_123456	Genomic	Automated	Genomic records that represent an assembly which does not reflect the structure of a real biological molecule. The assembly may represent an unordered assembly of unplaced scaffolds, or it may represent an assembly of DNA sequences generated from a biological sample that may not represent a single organism.

Exercise: 1

AIM: to retrieve a nucleotide sequence of Homo sapiens prostaglandin-endoperoxide synthase 1

Procedure

Login to NCBI web site: http://www.ncbi.nlm.nih.gov

Nucleotide was selected from the drop down menu in search input box.

Key word prostaglandin-endoperoxide synthase 1 is typed in "for" input box, and then Click go.

A list of search results related to keyword is obtained.

From the given list select the sequence of our interest i.e. prostaglandin-endoperoxide synthase 1 (NM_080591.1) was selected.

By clicking on the hyperlink the sequence entry form is displayed.

By Clicking FASTA on top, one can get the sequence in fasta format.

Result

The Nucleotide sequence of prostaglandin-endoperoxide synthase 1 of human(NM_080591.1) is obtained.

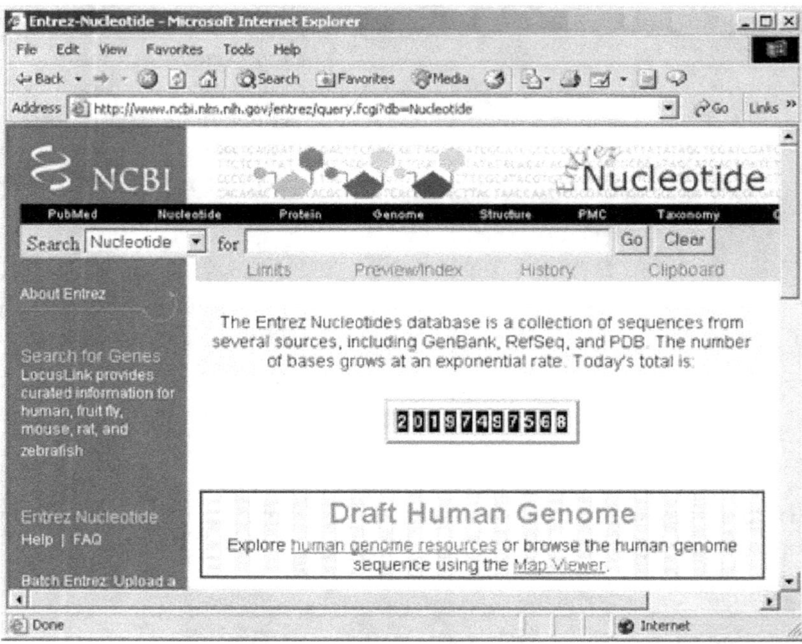

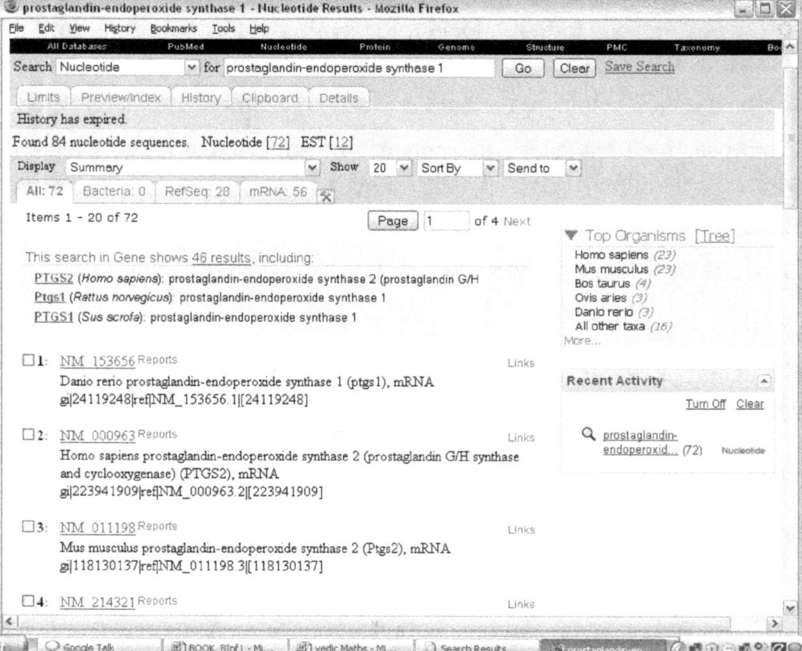

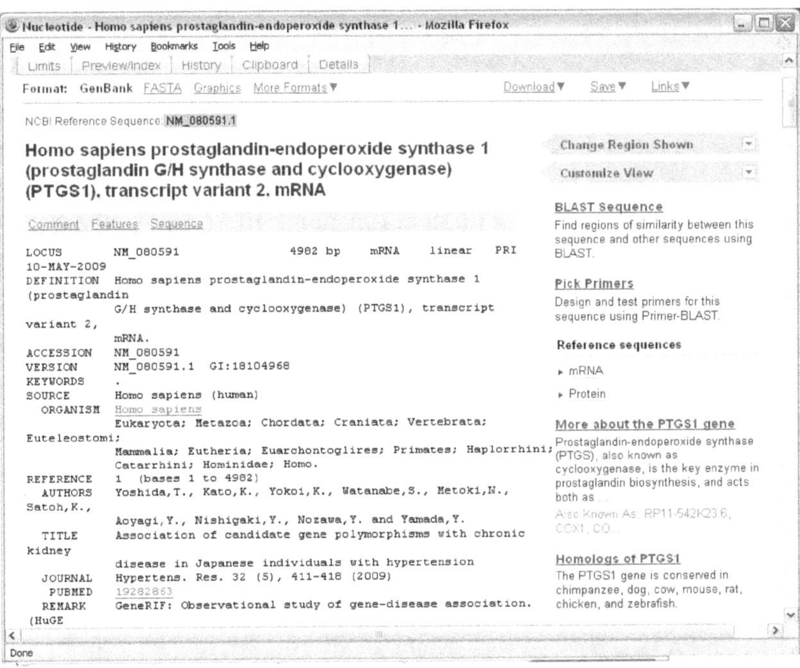

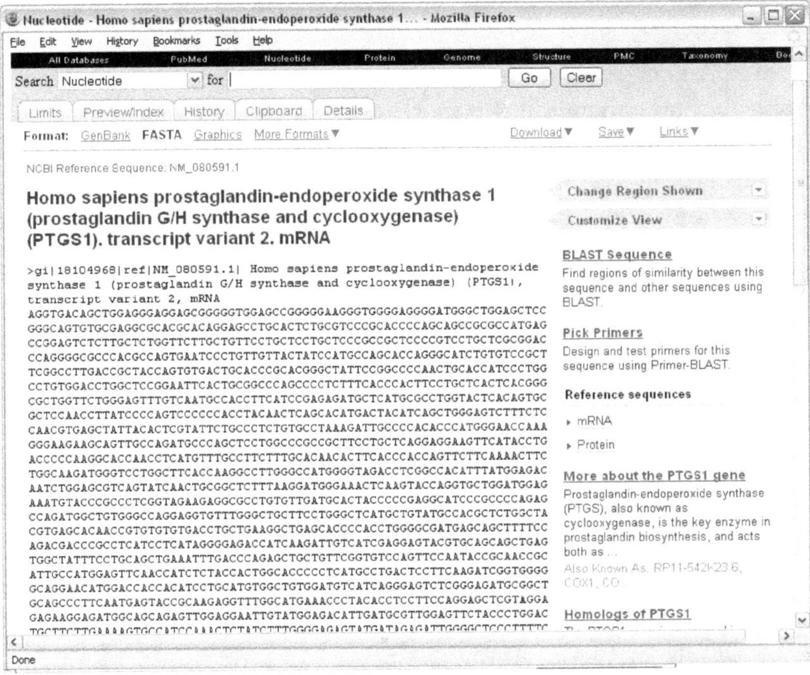

UniProtKB/Swiss – Prot The Protein sequence Database

UniProtKB/Swiss-Prot is a manually annotated protein knowledgebase established in 1986 and maintained since 2003 by the UniProt Consortium, a collaboration between the Swiss Institute of Bioinformatics (SIB) and the Department of Bioinformatics and Structural Biology of the Geneva University, the European Bioinformatics Institute (EBI) and the Georgetown University Medical Center's Protein Information Resource (PIR).

UniProtKB/Swiss-Prot, together with UniProtKB/TrEMBL, its computer-annotated supplement, constitutes the UniProt Knowledgebase (UniProtKB), a major project of the UniProt consortium. UniProtKB/Swiss-Prot and UniProtKB/TrEMBL give access to all the publicly available protein sequences.

The UniProt Knowledgebase consists of sequence entries. Sequence entries are composed of different line-types, each with their own format. For standardization purposes the format of the UniProt Knowledgebase follows as closely as possible that of the EMBL Nucleotide Sequence Database.

The UniProtKB/Swiss-Prot database distinguishes itself from other protein sequence databases by three distinct criteria:

1. Annotation

Data integrated into UniProtKB/Swiss-Prot, including the protein sequence and current knowledge on each protein, are manually checked and continuously updated. Each UniProtKB/Swiss-Prot entry contains core data (sequence data; bibliographical references and taxonomic data (description of the biological source of the protein)) and annotation, which consists of the description of the following items:

- Function(s) of the protein
- Post-translational modification(s). For example carbohydrates, phosphorylation, acetylation, GPI-anchor, etc.
- Domains and sites. For example calcium binding regions, ATP-binding sites, zinc fingers, homeobox, kringle, etc.
- Secondary structure
- Quaternary structure. For example homodimer, heterotrimer, etc.
- Similarities to other proteins
- Disease(s) associated with deficiencie(s) in the protein
- Sequence conflicts, variants, etc.

A special emphasis is laid on the annotation of biological events which generate protein diversity that cannot be predicted at the genomic level. Alternative products (alternative splicing), RNA editing and post-translational modifications (PTMs) are extensively annotated. For additional information, see Boeckmann et al., C.R.Biol. (2005) [16286078].

Our main sources of data are scientific publications, that report new sequence data, and/or review articles to periodically update the annotations of families or groups of proteins. We also make use of external experts, who have been recruited to send us their comments and updates concerning specific groups of proteins.

The annotation is mainly found in the comment lines (CC), in the feature table (FT) and in the keyword lines (KW). Most comments are classified by `topics'; this approach permits the easy retrieval of specific categories of data from the database.

2. Minimal redundancy

In order to have minimal redundancy and to improve sequence reliability, all protein sequences encoded by a same gene are merged into a single UniProtKB/Swiss-Prot entry. Differences found between various sequencing reports are analysed and fully described in the feature table (alternative splicing events, polymorphisms or conflicts for example).

3. Integration with other databases

Detailed expertise that goes behond the scope of UniProtKB/Swiss-Prot is made available via cross-references to specialised data collections such as EMBL/GenBank/DDBJ nucleotide sequence databases, 3D structure database (PDB), various protein domain and family characterisation databases etc. UniProtKB/Swiss-Prot is currently cross-referenced with about 60 different databases. Cross-references indicated in the DR lines are used to provide 'explicit' links to many databases; additionally, 'implicit' links are created on the fly by the ExPASy server.

Exercise: 2

Aim: To retrieve Human protein sequence information from UniProtKB/Swiss-Prot

Procedure

Login to http://www.expasy.ch/sprot/

Key word leptin is typed in "for" input box, then Click go.

A list of search results related to keyword is obtained.

From the given list select the sequence of our interest i.e Human leptin LEP_HUMAN(P41159) was selected.

By clicking on the hyperlink the sequence entry form is displayed.

Result

The protein sequence of leptin of human(P41159) is obtained.

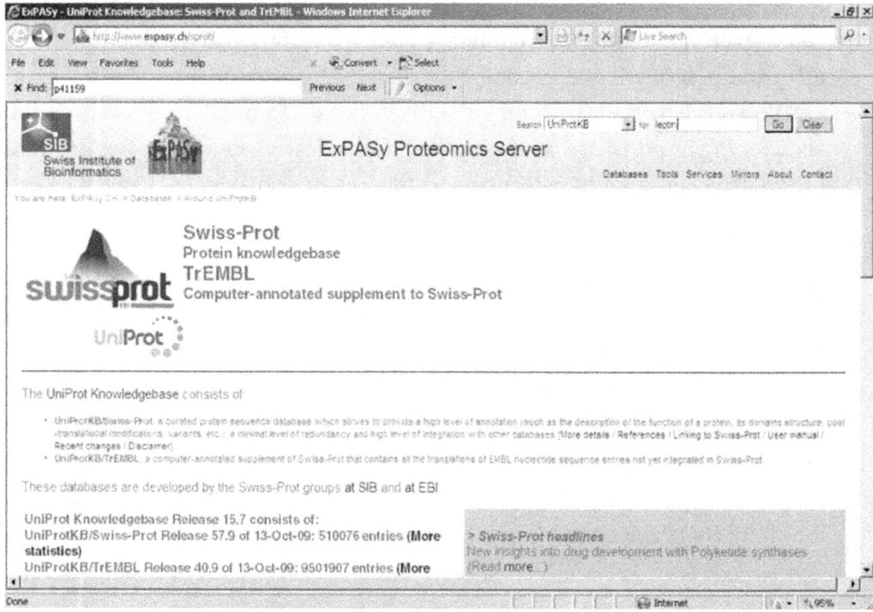

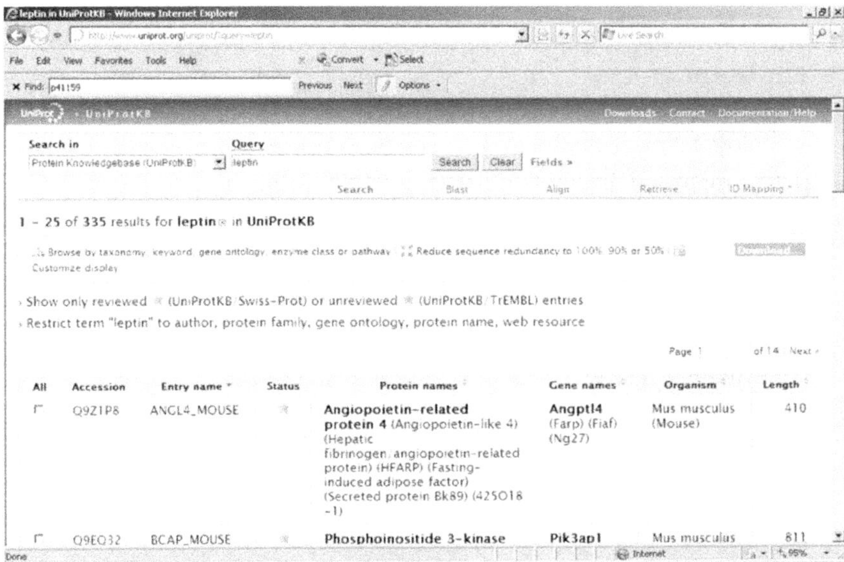

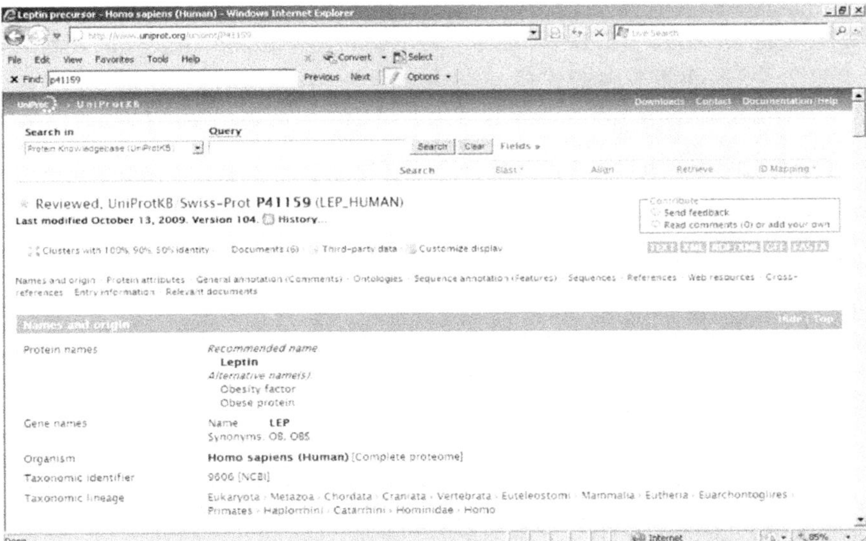

PDB – The Structural Database
Protein Databank

- Protein Data Bank is an international archive of 3D-structural information for Biological macromolecules.

- PDB is managed by the RCSB (Research Collaboratory for Structural Bioinformatics); an non-profit consortium involving rut gears, The State University of New Jersey; National Institute of Standards & Technology (NIST); and Saniego Supercomputer Centre and the University of California, SanDiego.

- Users can query the archive by PDB ID or keyword using the search box on the main page. Other query option include search (keyword search form with examples),search fields(and advanced search option with customizable fields),and status search (used to find structure being processed by PDB).

- Each structure records includes a summary .Structure viewing options, download and display options, links to records of structural neighbors, geometry, links to other protein information sources, and details about the structure sequence.

The data format of PDB file is well established and is widely recognized by almost all software designed to read and manipulate structural data, in some of the sequence databases

Like Gen Bank entry, every line in a PDB co-ordinate file begins with a word that identifies the type of information present in that line. These keyword or identifiers may be grouped into many sections viz. title, Primary structure, Heterogeneous, secondary structure, Crystallographic and co-ordinate transformations, co-ordinates and connectivity.

In the title section keywords point to information about the name, source etc, of the compound, details of authors, the references to published literature, and up to 1000 lines of general information about the structures, including all necessary experimental details required to interpret the structure contains keywords pointing to the protein or nucleic acid sequence of the structure in that file. References to sequence databases are also given here. Information on atoms that do not belong to the protein or nucleic acid, such as water, ions, and prosthetic groups is given under keywords that are classified as heterogeneous.

The section on the Secondary structure describes secondary structure features in the molecule. In particular, it specifies the positions of alpha helices, beta sheets and turns in the protein specifies tertiary interactions such as disulphide bonds, hydrogen bonds and salt bridges. The section on crystallographic and co-ordinate transformations is, of course, specific to crystallographic structures. Here we wish to transform the co-ordinate from that Cartesian axial system in which they occur in the Protein Data Bank to the crystallographic co-ordinate system in which they are specified in the original experimental structure determination. Such transformations are essential to study intermolecular interactions between any given molecule and its neighbour in crystal.

The most important part of the entry is specified by keywords in the co-ordinate section. Of these, the atomic co-ordinate of the molecule all begins with the word 'ATOM'. Each line that begins with 'ATOMS' has the co-ordinates of one atom of the molecule arranged in a very specific format. In fact it is this format commonly referred to as the PDB format. Each 'ATOM' record starts with an identifier of the atom that includes a serial number, atom name, residue name, polypeptide or nucleic acid chain name and residue name.

The Atom records are followed by the HETATM records that give the co-ordinates of the heteroatom in exactly the same format. After the terminator keyword 'TER' come the connectivity records that describe the bonds that connect the atoms to one another. This information is some time redundant since such information can always be calculated from the co-ordinates .If the distance between two atoms is less than the sum of their normal automatic radii, it is usually assumed that they are bonded, the nature of bond corresponding to that actual distance between the two. The file ends with the keyword 'END'.

Exercise: 3

PDB

Aim: To retrieve a protein structure of human obesity protein leptin. From protein databank.

Procedure :

Login to RCSB website: www.rcsb.org

Keyword leptin was typed in keyword search box.

A list of search results related to keyword was obtained.

From the list the structure detail of our interest was selected (1AX8).

By double clicking on the hyperlink the structure information was displayed.

To retrieve the pdb format file Select download file on the Rio side of the web page, and click pdb text.

Download the pdb file on to your system.

Result: The protein structure of leptin was retrived

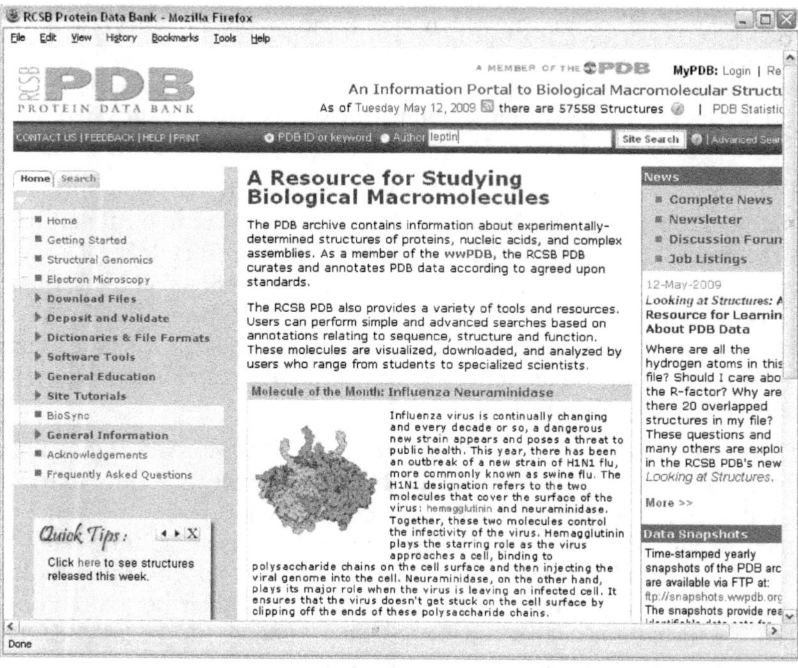

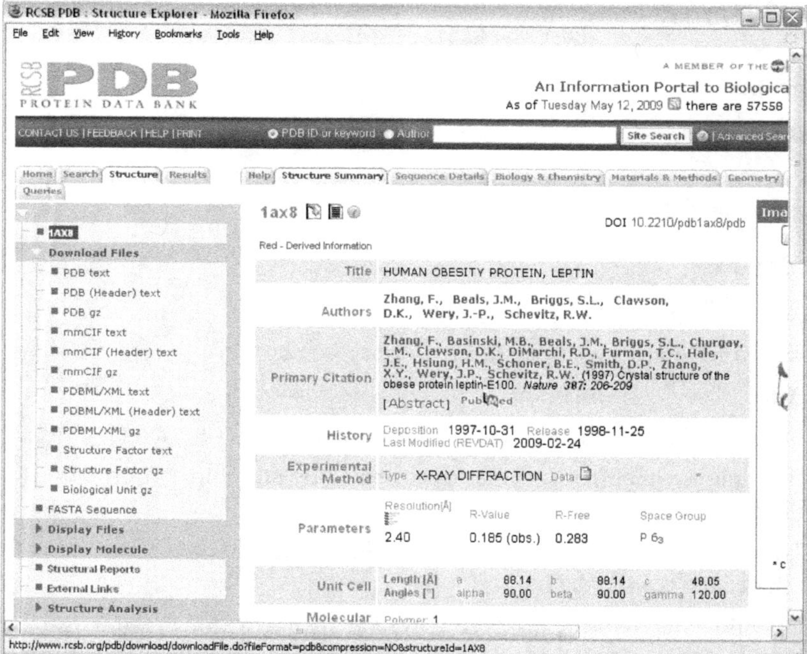

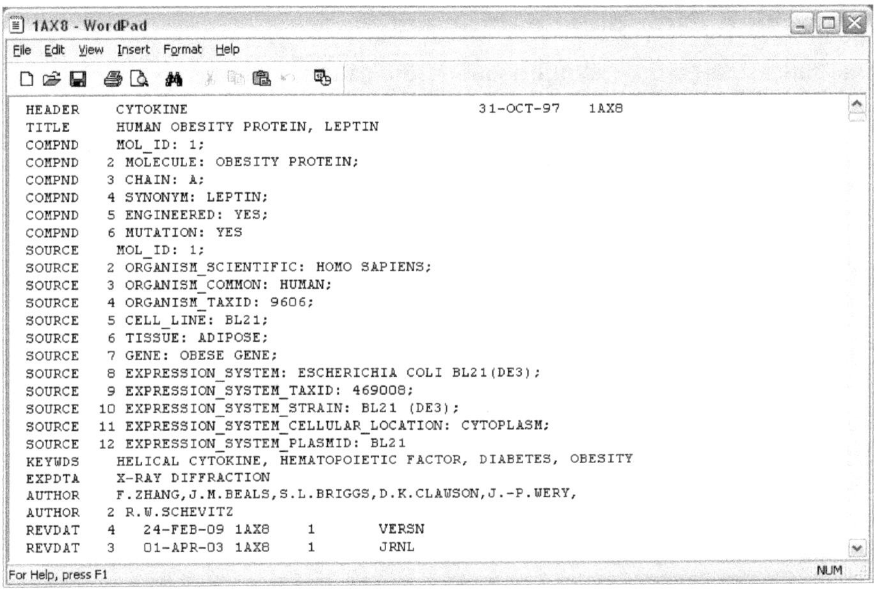

```
1AX8 - WordPad
File  Edit  View  Insert  Format  Help

HEADER    CYTOKINE                                31-OCT-97   1AX8
TITLE     HUMAN OBESITY PROTEIN, LEPTIN
COMPND    MOL_ID: 1;
COMPND    2 MOLECULE: OBESITY PROTEIN;
COMPND    3 CHAIN: A;
COMPND    4 SYNONYM: LEPTIN;
COMPND    5 ENGINEERED: YES;
COMPND    6 MUTATION: YES
SOURCE    MOL_ID: 1;
SOURCE    2 ORGANISM_SCIENTIFIC: HOMO SAPIENS;
SOURCE    3 ORGANISM_COMMON: HUMAN;
SOURCE    4 ORGANISM_TAXID: 9606;
SOURCE    5 CELL_LINE: BL21;
SOURCE    6 TISSUE: ADIPOSE;
SOURCE    7 GENE: OBESE GENE;
SOURCE    8 EXPRESSION_SYSTEM: ESCHERICHIA COLI BL21(DE3);
SOURCE    9 EXPRESSION_SYSTEM_TAXID: 469008;
SOURCE    10 EXPRESSION_SYSTEM_STRAIN: BL21 (DE3);
SOURCE    11 EXPRESSION_SYSTEM_CELLULAR_LOCATION: CYTOPLASM;
SOURCE    12 EXPRESSION_SYSTEM_PLASMID: BL21
KEYWDS    HELICAL CYTOKINE, HEMATOPOIETIC FACTOR, DIABETES, OBESITY
EXPDTA    X-RAY DIFFRACTION
AUTHOR    F.ZHANG,J.M.BEALS,S.L.BRIGGS,D.K.CLAWSON,J.-P.WERY,
AUTHOR    2 R.W.SCHEVITZ
REVDAT    4    24-FEB-09 1AX8    1        VERSN
REVDAT    3    01-APR-03 1AX8    1        JRNL

For Help, press F1                                          NUM
```

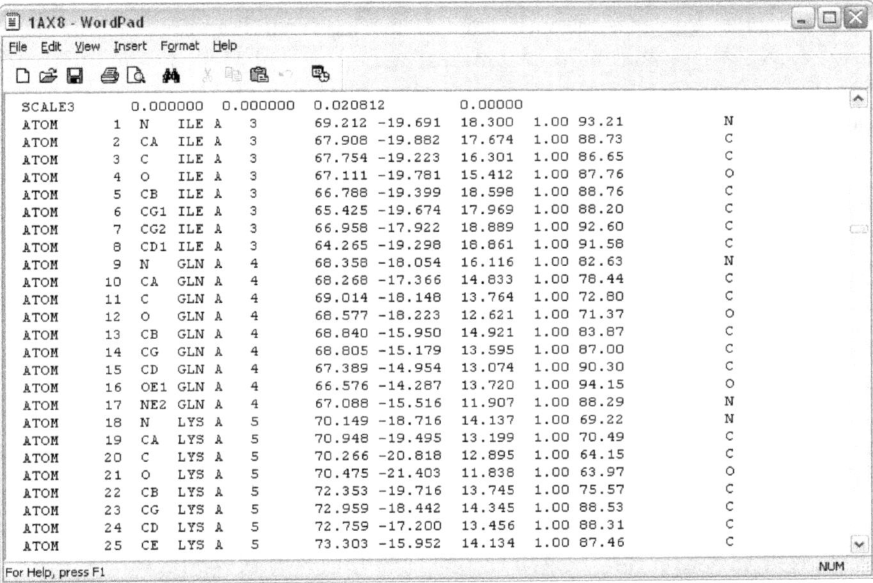

```
1AX8 - WordPad
File  Edit  View  Insert  Format  Help

SCALE3      0.000000  0.000000  0.020812     0.00000
ATOM     1  N   ILE A   3    69.212 -19.691  18.300  1.00 93.21      N
ATOM     2  CA  ILE A   3    67.908 -19.882  17.674  1.00 88.73      C
ATOM     3  C   ILE A   3    67.754 -19.223  16.301  1.00 86.65      C
ATOM     4  O   ILE A   3    67.111 -19.781  15.412  1.00 87.76      O
ATOM     5  CB  ILE A   3    66.788 -19.399  18.598  1.00 88.76      C
ATOM     6  CG1 ILE A   3    65.425 -19.674  17.969  1.00 88.20      C
ATOM     7  CG2 ILE A   3    66.958 -17.922  18.889  1.00 92.60      C
ATOM     8  CD1 ILE A   3    64.265 -19.298  18.861  1.00 91.58      C
ATOM     9  N   GLN A   4    68.358 -18.054  16.116  1.00 82.63      N
ATOM    10  CA  GLN A   4    68.268 -17.366  14.833  1.00 78.44      C
ATOM    11  C   GLN A   4    69.014 -18.148  13.764  1.00 72.80      C
ATOM    12  O   GLN A   4    68.577 -18.223  12.621  1.00 71.37      O
ATOM    13  CB  GLN A   4    68.840 -15.950  14.921  1.00 83.87      C
ATOM    14  CG  GLN A   4    68.805 -15.179  13.595  1.00 87.00      C
ATOM    15  CD  GLN A   4    67.389 -14.954  13.074  1.00 90.30      C
ATOM    16  OE1 GLN A   4    66.576 -14.287  13.720  1.00 94.15      O
ATOM    17  NE2 GLN A   4    67.088 -15.516  11.907  1.00 88.29      N
ATOM    18  N   LYS A   5    70.149 -18.716  14.137  1.00 69.22      N
ATOM    19  CA  LYS A   5    70.948 -19.495  13.199  1.00 70.49      C
ATOM    20  C   LYS A   5    70.266 -20.818  12.895  1.00 64.15      C
ATOM    21  O   LYS A   5    70.475 -21.403  11.838  1.00 63.97      O
ATOM    22  CB  LYS A   5    72.353 -19.716  13.745  1.00 75.57      C
ATOM    23  CG  LYS A   5    72.959 -18.442  14.345  1.00 88.53      C
ATOM    24  CD  LYS A   5    72.759 -17.200  13.456  1.00 88.31      C
ATOM    25  CE  LYS A   5    73.303 -15.952  14.134  1.00 87.46      C

For Help, press F1                                          NUM
```

Accessing Biological databases

One can access Biological information from databases through

Entrez

SRS-Sequence Retrieval System.

DBGET.

Entrez

The **Entrez** Global Query Cross-Database Search System is a powerful federated search engine, or web portal that allows users to search many discrete health sciences databases at the National Center for Biotechnology Information (NCBI) website. NCBI is part of the National Library of Medicine (NLM), itself a department of the National Institutes of Health (NIH) of the United States government. Entrez also happens to be the French second person plural (or formal) form of the verb "to enter", meaning literally "come in".

Entrez Global Query is an integrated search and retrieval system that provides access to all databases simultaneously with a single query string and user interface. *Entrez* is the integrated, text-based search and retrieval system used at NCBI for the major databases, including PubMed, Nucleotide and Protein Sequences, Protein Structures, Complete Genomes, Taxonomy, and others.

Entrez can efficiently retrieve related sequences, structures, and references. The Entrez system can provide views of gene and protein sequences and chromosome maps. Some textbooks are also available online through the Entrez system.

The Entrez front page provides, by default, access to the global query. All databases indexed by Entrez can be searched via a single query string, supporting Boolean operators and search term tags to limit parts of the search statement to particular fields. This returns a unified results page, that shows the number of hits for the search in each of the databases, which are also links to actual search results for that particular database.

Entrez also provides a similar interface for searching each particular database and for refining search results. The Limits feature allows the user to narrow a search a web forms interface. The History feature gives a numbered list of recently performed queries. Results of previous queries can be referred to by number and combined via boolean operators. Search results can be saved temporarily in a Clipboard. Users with a MyNCBI account can save queries indefinitely and also choose to have updates with new search results e-mailed for saved queries of most databases. It is widely used in the field of biotechnology to enhance the knowledge of students worldwide.

The Sequence Retrieval System (SRS) developed by Thure Etzold is a system for **integrating heterogenous databases**. It is based on premade indexes of the items (words, entries, data fields, text,...) found in a set of documents (database files). Apart from the database files themselves, the indexing procedure requires a grammar (Icarus) that describes what different words in the data files mean, how they are to be indexed, and how they cross-reference to other items in other databases. SRS is a web-oriented system located on a server which is accessed through HTML pages and CGI scripts.

SRS started as an academic project, but it is now a commercial system developed and marketed by LION Bioscience AG. However, academic groups can license the SRS system free of charge and set it up at a server in their own lab.

EBI runs an SRS service which can be used by anyone. It indexes a large number of databases, and it also provides a well-defined web interface which allows programs or web sites to create links that query SRS at EBI.

DBGET is an integrated database retrieval system for major biological databases, which are classified into five categories:

Category	Main commands			Remark
	bget	bfind	blink	
1. KEGG databases in DBGET	yes	yes	yes	Mirrored at GenomeNet
2. Other DBGET databases	yes	yes	yes	
3. Searchable databases on the Web	no	yes	yes	Used as Web resources
4. Link-only databases on the Web	no	no	yes	
5. PubMed database	yes	no	yes	

Databases in the third category are integrated for keyword seach, but the actual data are to be obtained from the original sites. Databases in the fourth category are available only in the LinkDB system. PubMed is a link-only database, but the bget page is generated using the NCBI service in order to better integrate with KEGG and other DBGET databases.

To access DBGET

http://www.genome.ad.jp/dbget/

http://www.genome.ad.jp/dbget-bin/www_bfind_sub?mode=bfind&max_hit=1000&dbkey=all&keywords=+prostaglandin-endoperoxide+synthase+1

2

Sequence Analysis

Biological Sequence Analysis

Usually, biologically motivated problems in computer science primarily involve sequences or strings. Examples of such problems are reconstruction of long strings of DNA from overlapping string fragments, comparing two or more strings for similarity. Searching of databases for related sequences and sub-sequences, looking for patterns or motifs in Bio-molecular sequences and more for all these, sequence comparison and alignment forms the basis. DNA, RNA and protein sequences are biological sequences.

Sequence alignment can be pair-wise alignment or multiple alignments. Pair-wise alignment is the process of comparing two strings. The simplest way of comparing two strings is to align them while trying to maximize matches, allowing for certain mismatches and inserting gap characters in either of the strings to bring them into a vertical register.

Pair-wise sequence alignment can be done in two ways

1. *Global alignment:* an alignment that covers the whole length of both sequences.
2. *Local alignment:* finds the best region of similarity between two sequences.

'Needleman and Wunsch algorithm' and 'Smith and Waterman algorithm' is used for performing global and local alignment respectively.

To access the quality of the alignment the alignments are given a score. Substitution matrices or scoring matrices like PAM & BLOSUM are used to score protein sequence alignment.

Multiple string comparison is a tool for abstracting and representing biological important commonalities from a set of strings. These commonalities may reveal evolutionary history, critical conserved motif, common 2 or 3 dimensional molecular structures or clues about the common biological functions of the strings. Such commonalities are used to characterize the families or super families of proteins. These characteristics are then used in database searches to identify other potential members of the family. When considering a protein for membership in an established family, it is more effective to align the candidate string, to a representation of the individual family members. One central technique for multiple string comparison involves multiple sequence alignment.There are several tools for alignment, for example, ClustalW which is the most popular, PROBCONS, MUSCLE, MAFFT, DIALIGN, T-Coffee, POA and MANGO.

Exercise: 4

LOCAL ALIGNMENT

Aim: To perform local alignment between the following sequences

Seq1:

>gi|6321538|ref|NP_011615.1| Mitochondrial serine protease required for the processing of various mitochondrial proteins and maintenance of mitochondrial DNA and morphology; belongs to the rhomboid-GlpG superfamily of intramembrane peptidases; Pcp1p [Saccharomyces cerevisiae]

MSGVSSVMLGLRPATRIFFRSNISVSPSRTFVSYIGRSQSTSILKNAPNLEDNVTNLQKI
IPKRFFSQTSILKSRWKPIFNEETTNRYVRLNRFQQYQQQRSGGNPLGSMTILGLSLMAG
IYFGSPYLFEHVPPFTYFKTHPKNLVYALLGINVAVFGLWQLPKCWRFLQKYMLLQKDYV
TSKISIIGSAFSHQEFWHLGMNMLALWSFGTSLATMLGASNFFSLYMNSAIAGSLFSLWY
PKLARLAIVGPSLGASGALFGVLGCFSYLFPHAKILLFVFPVPGGAWVAFLASVAWNAAG
CALRWGSFDYAAHLGGSMMGVLYGWYISKAVEKQRQRRLQAAGRWF

Seq2:

>sp|P48740|MASP1_HUMAN Complement-activating component of Ra-reactive factor OS=Homo sapiens GN=MASP1 PE=2 SV=2
MRWLLLYYALCFSLSKASAHTVELNNMFGQIQSPGYPDSYPSDSEVTWNITVPDGFRIKL
YFMHFNLESSYLCEYDYVKVETEDQVLATFCGRETTDTEQTPGQEVVLSPGSFMSITFRS
DFSNEERFTGFDAHYMAVDVDECKEREDEELSCDHYCHNYIGGYYCSCRFGYILHTDNRT
CRVECSDNLFTQRTGVITSPDFPNPYPKSSECLYTIELEEGFMVNLQFEDIFDIQDHPEV
PCPYDYIKIKVGPKVLGPFCGEKAPEPISTQSHSVLILFHSDNSAENRGWRLSYRAAGNE
CPELQPPVHGKIEPSQAKYFFKDQVLVSCDTGYKVLKDNVEMDTFQIECLKDGTWSNKIP
TCKIVDCRAPGELEHGLITFSTRNNLTTYKSEIKYSCQEPYYKMLNNNTGIYTCSAQGVW
MNKVLGRSLPTCLPVCGLPKFSRKLMARIFNGRPAQKGTTPWIAMLSHLNGQPFCGGSLL
GSSWIVTAAHCLHQSLDPKDPTLRDSDLLSPSDFKIILGKHWRLRSDENEQHLGVKHTTL
HPQYDPNTFENDVALVELLESPVLNAFVMPICLPEGPQQEGAMVIVSGWGKQFLQRFPET
LMEIEIPIVDHSTCQKAYAPLKKKVTRDMICAGEKEGGKDACAGDSGGPMVTLNRERGQW
YLVGTVSWGDDCGKKDRYGVYSYIHHNKDWIQRVTGVRN

Procedure:

Respective Protein sequences in fasta format of human and yeast were obtained by accessing Protein sequence databases (swissprot).

Log in to http://www.ebi.ac.uk/Tools/emboss/align/

Paste the respective sequences in the given input boxes.

Keep the method in water tool and remaining option buttons in default, click run.

Results were displayed as soon as the task completed.

Result:

The results show that 238 to 330 of yeast protein sequence locally aligned with human protein sequence from 419-489, with 23.1 idenity (indicated by double dots:) and 35.6 similarity(it includes both : & .).

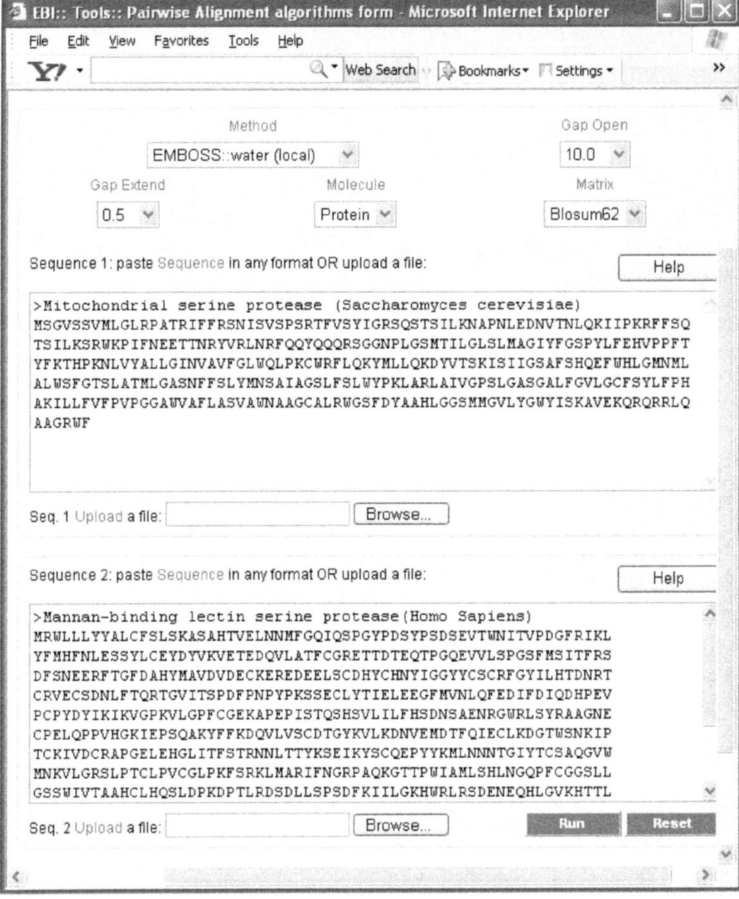

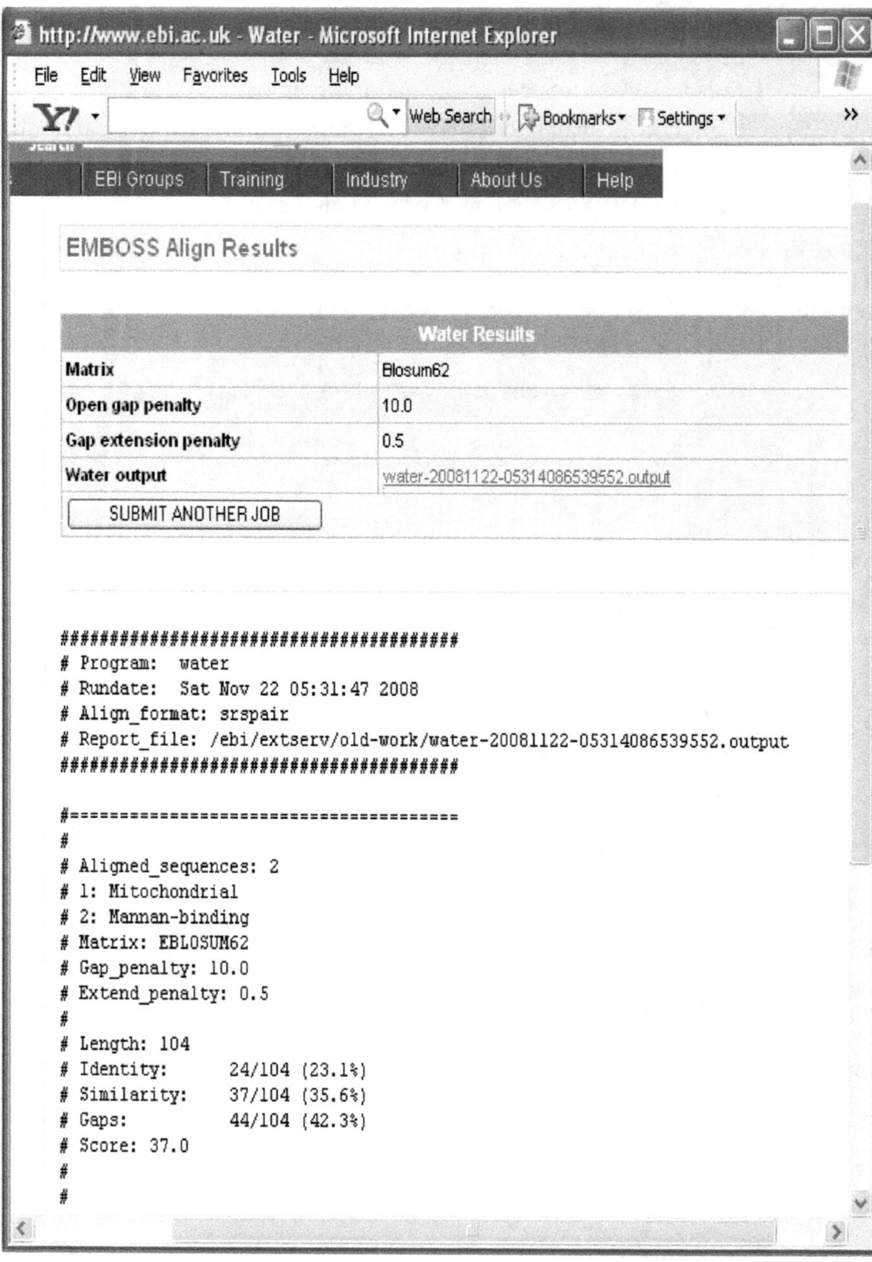

Water Results	
Matrix	Blosum62
Open gap penalty	10.0
Gap extension penalty	0.5
Water output	water-20081122-05314086539552.output


```
#######################################
# Program:  water
# Rundate:  Sat Nov 22 05:31:47 2008
# Align_format: srspair
# Report_file: /ebi/extserv/old-work/water-20081122-05314086539552.output
#######################################

#=======================================
#
# Aligned_sequences: 2
# 1: Mitochondrial
# 2: Mannan-binding
# Matrix: EBLOSUM62
# Gap_penalty: 10.0
# Extend_penalty: 0.5
#
# Length: 104
# Identity:      24/104 (23.1%)
# Similarity:    37/104 (35.6%)
# Gaps:          44/104 (42.3%)
# Score: 37.0
#
#
```

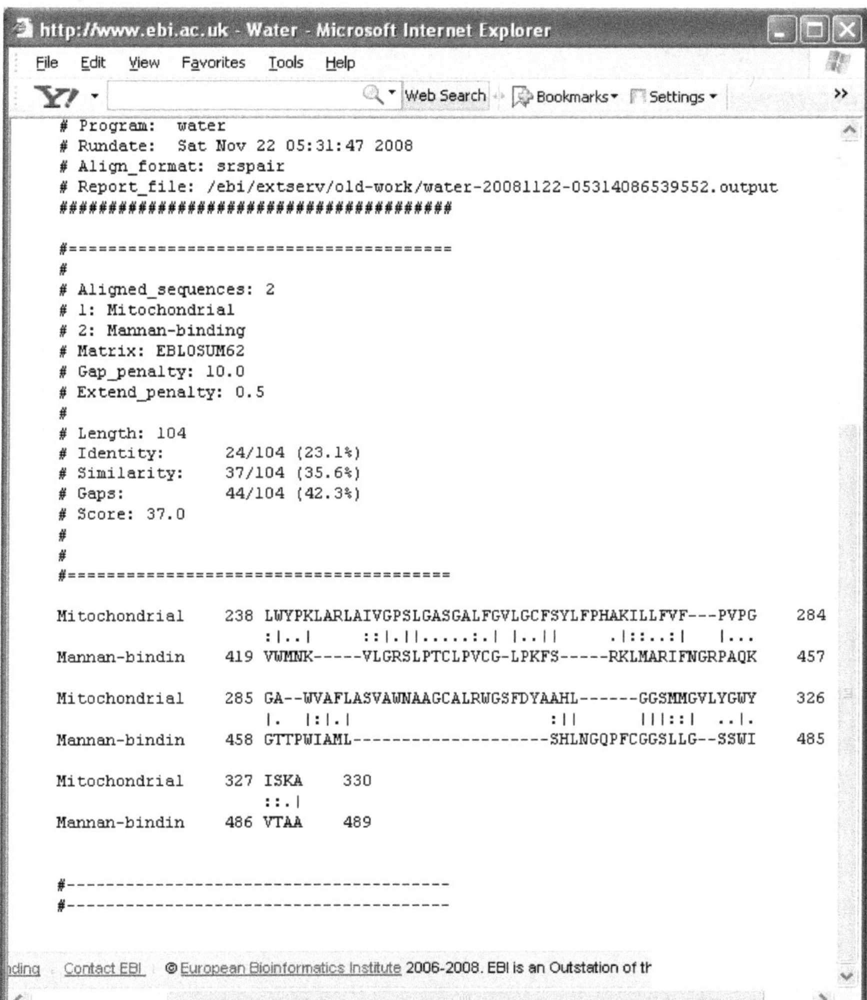


```
# Program:  water
# Rundate:  Sat Nov 22 05:31:47 2008
# Align_format: srspair
# Report_file: /ebi/extserv/old-work/water-20081122-05314086539552.output
########################################

#=======================================
#
# Aligned_sequences: 2
# 1: Mitochondrial
# 2: Mannan-binding
# Matrix: EBLOSUM62
# Gap_penalty: 10.0
# Extend_penalty: 0.5
#
# Length: 104
# Identity:     24/104 (23.1%)
# Similarity:   37/104 (35.6%)
# Gaps:         44/104 (42.3%)
# Score: 37.0
#
#
#=======================================

Mitochondrial    238 LWYPKLARLAIVGPSLGASGALFGVLGCFSYLFPHAKILLFVF---PVPG    284
                     :|..|       ::|.||.....:.| |..||    .|::..:|   |...
Mannan-bindin    419 VWMNK-----VLGRSLPTCLPVCG-LPKFS-----RKLMARIFNGRPAQK    457

Mitochondrial    285 GA--WVAFLASVAWNAAGCALRWGSFDYAAHL------GGSMMGVLYGWY    326
                     |.  |:|.|                      :||      |||::|  ..|.
Mannan-bindin    458 GTTPWIAML-------------------SHLNGQPFCGGSLLG--SSWI    485

Mitochondrial    327 ISKA     330
                     ::.|
Mannan-bindin    486 VTAA     489


#---------------------------------------
#---------------------------------------
```

Exercise: 5

Global Alignment

Aim: To perform global alignment between the following sequences

SEQ1

```
>gi|150393488|ref|YP_001316163.1| globin [Staphylococcus
aureus subsp. aureus JH1]
```

```
MTTTPYDIIGKEALYDMIDYFYTLVEKDERLNHLFPGDFAETSRKQKQFLTQFLGGPNIY
TEEHGHPMLRKRHMDFTITEFERDAWLENMQTAINRAAFPQGVGDYLFERLRLTANHMVN
S
```

SEQ2

```
>gi|57637203|gb|AAW53991.1| protozoan/cyanobacterial  globin
family protein [Staphylococcus epidermidis RP62A]
```

```
MSIRQITFKCKNSCYIRYILMEHGDIMSKTPYELIGQKALYQMIDHFYQLVEKDSRINHL
FPGDFKETSRKQKQFLTQFLGGPDLYTQEHGHPMLKRRHMEFTISEYERDAWLENMHTAI
QHAELPAGVGDYLFERLRLTAHHMVNS
```

Procedure

Respective Protein sequences in fasta format of human and yeast were obtained by accessing Protein sequence databases.

Log in to http://www.ebi.ac.uk/Tools/emboss/align/

Paste the respective sequences in the given input boxes.

Keep the method in Needle tool and remaining option buttons in default, click run.

Results were displayed as soon as the task completed.

Result

The results show that's 1 to 121 of S.aureus protein sequence globaly aligned with S.epedermidis protein sequence from 1-147, with 63.9% idenity (indicated by double dots:) and 74.8% similarity (it includes both : & .).

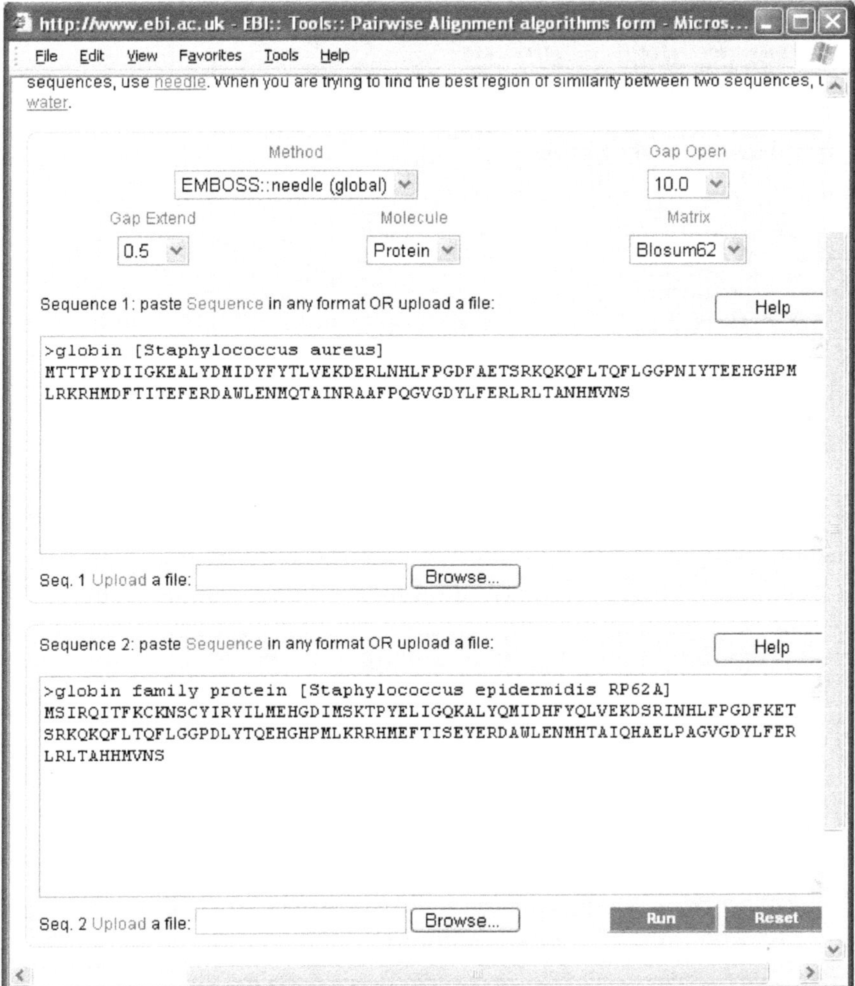

http://www.ebi.ac.uk - EBI:: Tools:: Pairwise Alignment algorithms form - Micros...
File   Edit   View   Favorites   Tools   Help
sequences, use needle. When you are trying to find the best region of similarity between two sequences, u
water.
Method
EMBOSS::needle (global)
Gap Open
10.0
Gap Extend
0.5
Molecule
Protein
Matrix
Blosum62
Sequence 1: paste Sequence in any format OR upload a file:
Help
>globin [Staphylococcus aureus]
MTTTPYDIIGKEALYDMIDYFYTLVEKDERLNHLFPGDFAETSRKQKQFLTQFLGGPNIYTEEHGHPM
LRKRHMDFTITEFERDAWLENMQTAINRAAFPQGVGDYLFERLRLTANHMVNS
Seq. 1 Upload a file: Browse...
Sequence 2: paste Sequence in any format OR upload a file:
Help
>globin family protein [Staphylococcus epidermidis RP62A]
MSIRQITFKCKNSCYIRYILMEHGDIMSKTPYELIGQKALYQMIDHFYQLVEKDSRINHLFPGDFKET
SRKQKQFLTQFLGGPDLYTQEHGHPMLKRRHMEFTISEYERDAWLENMHTAIQHAELPAGVGDYLFER
LRLTAHHMVNS
Seq. 2 Upload a file: Browse...   Run   Reset

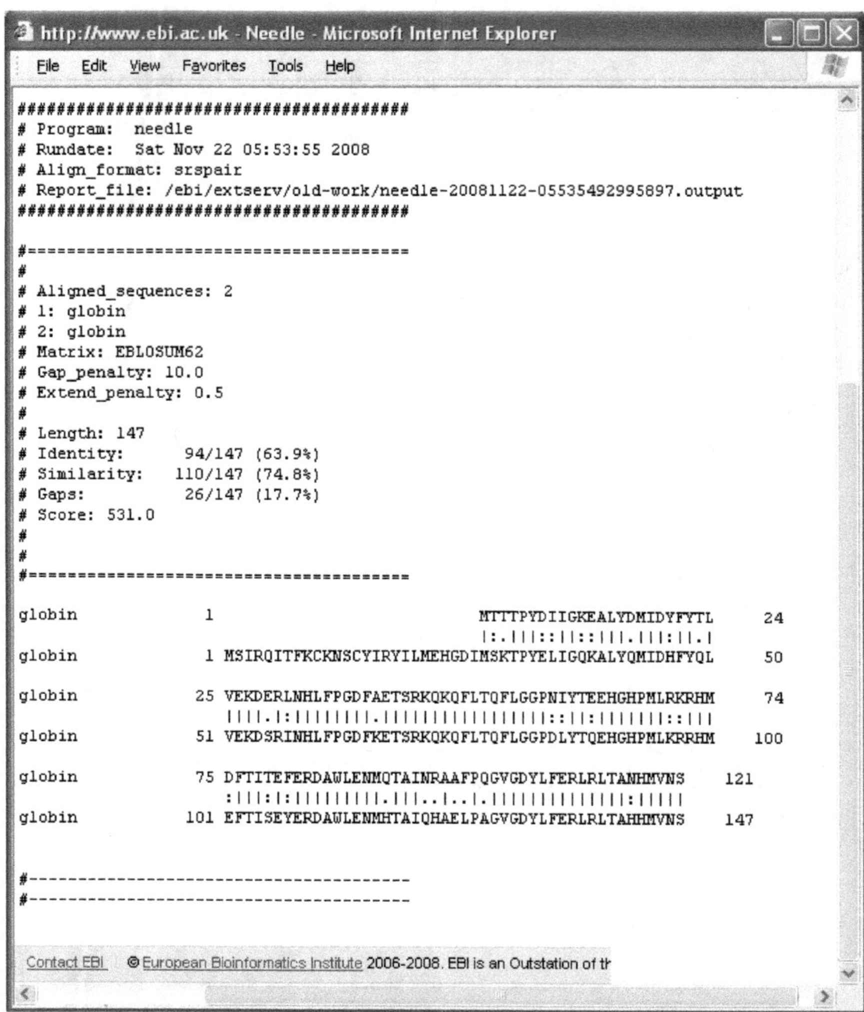


```
#######################################
# Program:  needle
# Rundate:  Sat Nov 22 05:53:55 2008
# Align_format: srspair
# Report_file: /ebi/extserv/old-work/needle-20081122-05535492995897.output
#######################################

#=======================================
#
# Aligned_sequences: 2
# 1: globin
# 2: globin
# Matrix: EBLOSUM62
# Gap_penalty: 10.0
# Extend_penalty: 0.5
#
# Length: 147
# Identity:      94/147 (63.9%)
# Similarity:   110/147 (74.8%)
# Gaps:          26/147 (17.7%)
# Score: 531.0
#
#
#=======================================

globin            1                         MTTTPYDIIGKEALYDMIDYFYTL     24
                                             |:.|||::||::|||.|||:||.|
globin            1 MSIRQITFKCKNSCYIRYILMEHGDIMSKTPYELIGQKALYQMIDHFYQL     50

globin           25 VEKDERLNHLFPGDFAETSRKQKQFLTQFLGGPNIYTEEHGHPMLRKRHM     74
                      ||||.|:|||||||||.|||||||||||||||||::||:||||||||::|||
globin           51 VEKDSRINHLFPGDFKETSRKQKQFLTQFLGGPDLYTQEHGHPMLKRRHM    100

globin           75 DFTITEFERDAWLENMQTAINRAAFPQGVGDYLFERLRLTANHMVNS    121
                      :|||:|:||||||||.|||..|...|.||||||||||||||:|||||
globin          101 EFTISEYERDAWLENMHTAIQHAELPAGVGDYLFERLRLTAHHMVNS    147


#---------------------------------------
#---------------------------------------
```

Exercise: 6

Multiple Sequence Alignment

Aim: To perform Multiple alignment between the following sequences

SEQ1

>gi|44955888|ref|NP_976312.1| myoglobin [Homo sapiens]

MGLSDGEWQLVLNVWGKVEADIPGHGQEVLIRLFKGHPETLEKFDKFKHLKSEDEMKASE
DLKKHGATVLTALGGILKKKGHHEAEIKPLAQSHATKHKIPVKYLEFISECIIQVLQSKH
PGDFGADAQGAMNKALELFRKDMASNYKELGFQG

SEQ2

>gi|21359820|ref|NP_038621.2| myoglobin [Mus musculus]
MGLSDGEWQLVLNVWGKVEADLAGHGQEVLIGLFKTHPETLDKFDKFKNLKSEEDMKGSE
DLKKHGCTVLTALGTILKKKGQHAAEIQPLAQSHATKHKIPVKYLEFISEIIIEVLKKRH
SGDFGADAQGAMSKALELFRNDIAAKYKELGFQG

SEQ3

>gi|11024650|ref|NP_067599.1| myoglobin [Rattus norvegicus]
MGLSDGEWQMVLNIWGKVEGDLAGHGQEVLISLFKAHPETLEKFDKFKNLKSEEEMKSSE
DLKKHGCTVLTALGTILKKKGQHAAEIQPLAQSHATKHKIPVKYLEFISEVIIQVLKKRY
SGDFGADAQGAMSKALELFRNDIAAKYKELGFQG

SEQ4

>gi|27806939|ref|NP_776306.1| myoglobin [Bos taurus]
MGLSDGEWQLVLNAWGKVEADVAGHGQEVLIRLFTGHPETLEKFDKFKHLKTEAEMKASE
DLKKHGNTVLTALGGILKKKGHHEAEVKHLAESHANKHKIPVKYLEFISDAIIHVLHAKH
PSDFGADAQAAMSKALELFRNDMAAQYKVLGFHG

Procedure

Respective Protein sequences in fasta format of human and yeast were obtained by accessing Protein sequence databases.

Log in to http://www.ebi.ac.uk/Tools/clustalw2/

Paste the respective sequences in the given input box.

Keep all the methods in default, click run.

Results were displayed as soon as the task completed.

Result

The results show that homosapiens are more related to cow (84% similarity) than mouse and rat (with 83 as score). Similarly mouse and rat more similar compare to human than cow.

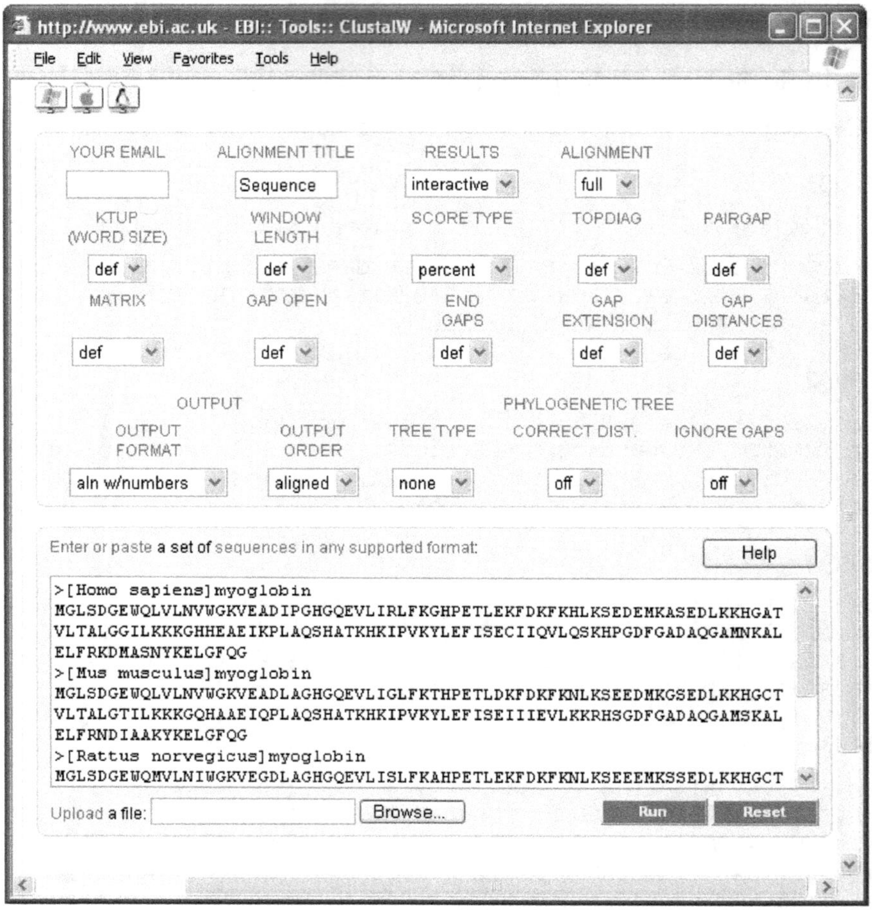

http://www.ebi.ac.uk - EBI:: Tools:: ClustalW - Microsoft Internet Explorer
File   Edit   View   Favorites   Tools   Help
YOUR EMAIL   ALIGNMENT TITLE   RESULTS   ALIGNMENT
                  Sequence   interactive   full
KTUP   WINDOW   SCORE TYPE   TOPDIAG   PAIRGAP
(WORD SIZE)   LENGTH
def   def   percent   def   def
MATRIX   GAP OPEN   END   GAP   GAP
                                         GAPS   EXTENSION   DISTANCES
def   def   def   def   def
OUTPUT   PHYLOGENETIC TREE
OUTPUT   OUTPUT   TREE TYPE   CORRECT DIST.   IGNORE GAPS
FORMAT   ORDER
aln w/numbers   aligned   none   off   off
Enter or paste a set of sequences in any supported format: Help
>[Homo sapiens]myoglobin
MGLSDGEWQLVLNVWGKVEADIPGHGQEVLIRLFKGHPETLEKFDKFKHLKSEDEMKASEDLKKHGAT
VLTALGGILKKKGHHEAEIKPLAQSHATKHKIPVKYLEFISECIIQVLQSKHPGDFGADAQGAMNKAL
ELFRKDMASNYKELGFQG
>[Mus musculus]myoglobin
MGLSDGEWQLVLNVWGKVEADLAGHGQEVLIGLFKTHPETLDKFDKFKNLKSEEDMKGSEDLKKHGCT
VLTALGTILKKKGQHAAEIQPLAQSHATKHKIPVKYLEFISEIIIEVLKKRHSGDFGADAQGAMSKAL
ELFRNDIAAKYKELGFQG
>[Rattus norvegicus]myoglobin
MGLSDGEWQMVLNIWGKVEGDLAGHGQEVLISLFKAHPETLEKFDKFKNLKSEEEMKSSEDLKKHGCT
Upload a file: Browse...   Run   Reset

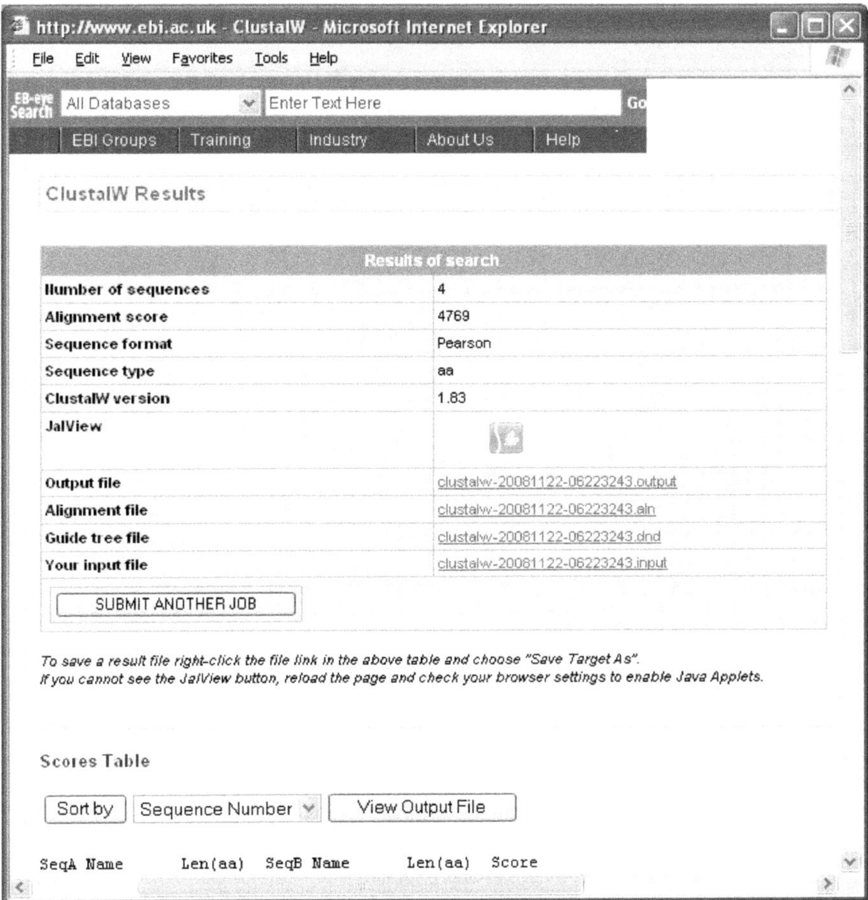
http://www.ebi.ac.uk - ClustalW - Microsoft Internet Explorer
File   Edit   View   Favorites   Tools   Help
EB-eye Search   All Databases   Enter Text Here   Go
EBI Groups   Training   Industry   About Us   Help
ClustalW Results
Results of search
Number of sequences   4
Alignment score   4769
Sequence format   Pearson
Sequence type   aa
ClustalW version   1.83
JalView
Output file   clustalw-20081122-06223243.output
Alignment file   clustalw-20081122-06223243.aln
Guide tree file   clustalw-20081122-06223243.dnd
Your input file   clustalw-20081122-06223243.input
SUBMIT ANOTHER JOB
To save a result file right-click the file link in the above table and choose "Save Target As".
If you cannot see the JalView button, reload the page and check your browser settings to enable Java Applets.
Scores Table
Sort by   Sequence Number   View Output File
SeqA Name   Len(aa)   SeqB Name   Len(aa)   Score

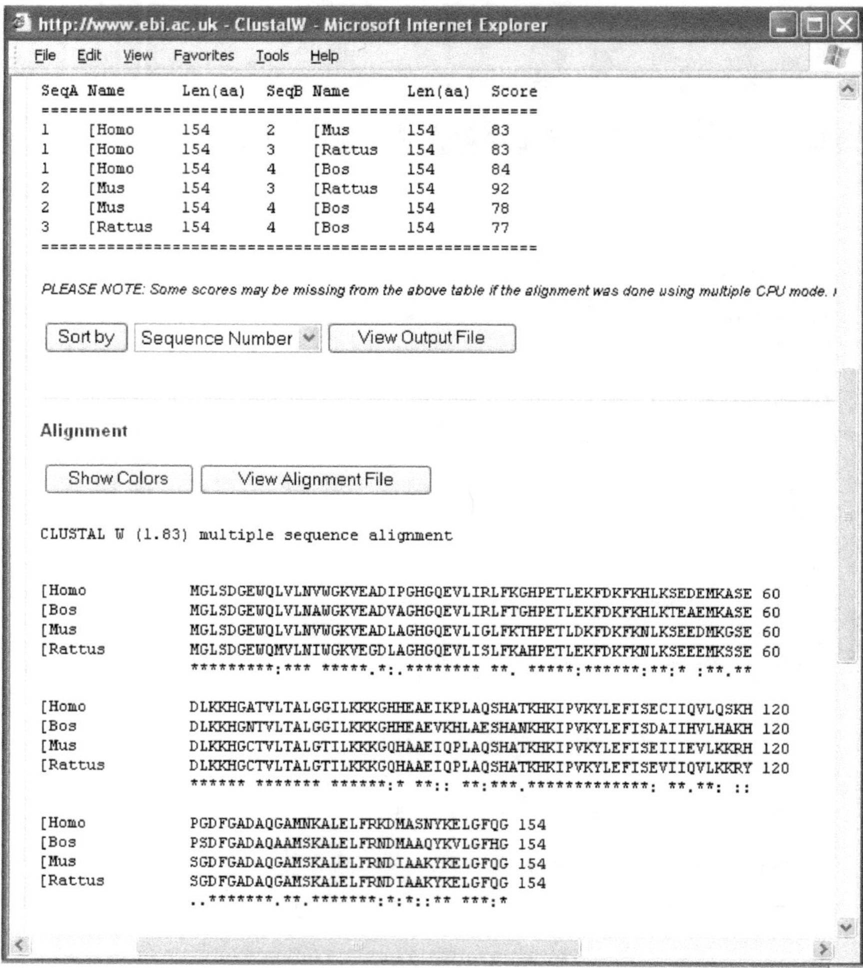

http://www.ebi.ac.uk - ClustalW - Microsoft Internet Explorer
File   Edit   View   Favorites   Tools   Help

SeqA Name   Len(aa) SeqB Name   Len(aa) Score
===
1   [Homo   154   2   [Mus   154   83
1   [Homo   154   3   [Rattus   154   83
1   [Homo   154   4   [Bos   154   84
2   [Mus   154   3   [Rattus   154   92
2   [Mus   154   4   [Bos   154   78
3   [Rattus   154   4   [Bos   154   77
===

PLEASE NOTE: Some scores may be missing from the above table if the alignment was done using multiple CPU mode.

Sort by   Sequence Number   View Output File

Alignment

Show Colors   View Alignment File

CLUSTAL W (1.83) multiple sequence alignment

[Homo   MGLSDGEWQLVLNVWGKVEADIPGHGQEVLIRLFKGHPETLEKFDKFKHLKSEDEMKASE 60
[Bos   MGLSDGEWQLVLNAWGKVEADVAGHGQEVLIRLFTGHPETLEKFDKFKHLKTEAEMKASE 60
[Mus   MGLSDGEWQLVLNVWGKVEADLAGHGQEVLIGLFKTHPETLDKFDKFKNLKSEEDMKGSE 60
[Rattus   MGLSDGEWQMVLNIWGKVEGDLAGHGQEVLISLFKAHPETLEKFDKFKNLKSEEEMKSSE 60
               ********:*** *****.*:.******* **. *****:******:**:* :**.**

[Homo   DLKKHGATVLTALGGILKKKGHHEAEIKPLAQSHATKHKIPVKYLEFISECIIQVLQSKH 120
[Bos   DLKKHGNTVLTALGGILKKKGHHEAEVKHLAESHANKHKIPVKYLEFISDAIIHVLHAKH 120
[Mus   DLKKHGCTVLTALGTILKKKGQHAAEIQPLAQSHATKHKIPVKYLEFISEIIIEVLKKRH 120
[Rattus   DLKKHGCTVLTALGTILKKKGQHAAEIQPLAQSHATKHKIPVKYLEFISEVIIQVLKKRY 120
               ****** ******* ******:* **:: **:***.*************: **.**: ::

[Homo   PGDFGADAQGAMNKALELFRKDMASNYKELGFQG 154
[Bos   PSDFGADAQAAMSKALELFRNDMAAQYKVLGFHG 154
[Mus   SGDFGADAQGAMSKALELFRNDIAAKYKELGFQG 154
[Rattus   SGDFGADAQGAMSKALELFRNDIAAKYKELGFQG 154
               ..*******.**.*******:*:*::** ***:*

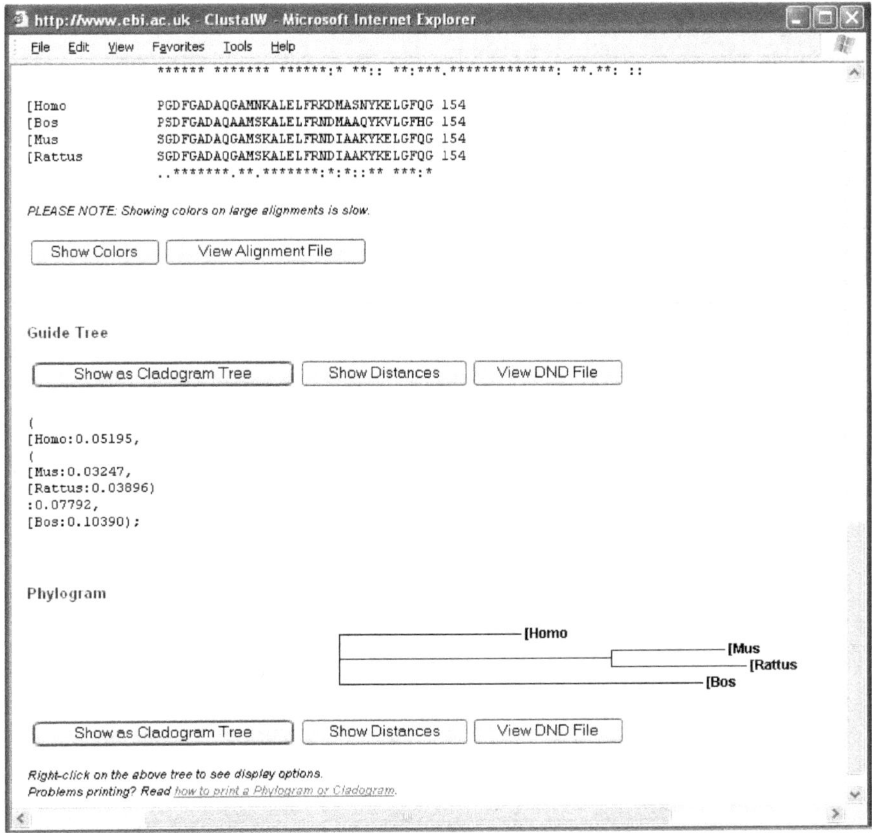

SIMILARITY SEARCH TOOLS- BLAST

BLAST

➢ **BLAST** stands for **Basic Local Alignment Search Tool.**

➢ It is a similarity search tool available at **National Centre for Biotechnology Information NCBI, USA.**

➢ It is a heuristics based algorithm.

➢ It is a word based method and requires a preformatted search database.

➢ It initially finds the list of high scoring words (w). BLAST takes each word from the query sequence and locates all the words in the current test sequence.

  E.g. *w is 3 for amino acid sequence and 11 for the nucleotide sequence*

> Compare the word list to the database and identify the exact matches. If similar words are found BLAST tries to expand the alignment to the adjacent words without allowing the gaps.

> After all words are tested, a set of maximal segment pairs is chosen for the database sequence.

BLAST OUTPUT

> BLAST output includes the graphical overview box, a matching list and a text description of the alignment.

> The graphical overview box contains colored horizontal bars that allow quick identification of the number of database hits and the degree of similarity of the hits.

> The color coding of the horizontal bars corresponds to ranking of similarities of the sequence hits.

Red color – high similarity

Green and blue – moderately related

Black – less similar

> The length of the bars represents the spans of sequence alignments relative to the query sequence. Each bar is hyperlinked to the actual pair wise alignment in the text portion of the report.

> Below the graphical box is a list of matching hits ranked by E-values in ascending order. Each hit includes the accession number, title of the database record, bit score and E-value. This list is followed by the text description which may be divided into 3 sections. First one is header. This section contains the gene index number or the reference number of the database hit and the one-line description of the database sequence. Second section is statistics. This includes the bit score, E-value, percentages of identity, similarity and gaps. Third section is alignment. In this section, the query sequence is on the top of the pair and the database sequence is at the bottom of the pair labeled as subject.

> In between the two sequences matching identical residues are written out at their corresponding position whereas non-identical but similar residues are labeled with plus mark (+).

> Any residues identified as low complexity regions (LCRs) in the query sequence are masked with Xs and Ns so that no adjustment is represented in those regions.

Statistical significance of BLAST

BLAST output provides a list of pair-wise sequence matches ranked by statistical significance. The significant scores help to distinguish evolutionary related sequences from unrelated ones. In BLAST searches, this statistical indicator is known as E-values (Expectation value). It indicates the probability that the resulting alignments from a database search are caused by random chance.

$$E = m*n*p$$

m = total number of residues in a database

n = number of residues in the query sequence

p = probability that an hsp alignment is the result of random chance

E-value is related to the p-value which is used to assess significance of single pair wise alignment. This E-value provides information about the likelihood that given sequence's match is purely by chance.

If E-value<1e-50 it is considered that the database match is the result of homologous relationship.

If E is between 0.01 and 1e-50 match is considered homology.

If E is between 0.01 and 10 match is considered not significant

If E>10 it's considered as a distant relationship.

Blast Program Options

PROGRAM	QUERY SEQUENCE	DATABASE	TYPE OF ALIGNMENT
BLASTP	Protein	Protein	Gapped
BLASTn	Nucleic acid	Nucleic acid	Gapped
BLAST x	Translated nucleic acids	Protein	Each frame gapped
T BLAST n	Protein	Translated nucleic acids	Each frame gapped
T BLAST x	Translated nucleic acids	Translated nucleic acid	Each frame gapped

Exercise: 7

Aim: To perform BLASTp against pdb database.

Query sequence – P71913

Procedure:

1. The Ribokinase protein of mycobacterium tuberculosis sequence was selected from the database.
2. login to http://blast.ncbi.nlm.nih.gov/Blast.cgi
3. Select the BlastP as the input sequence is protein.
4. Paste the protein sequence in fasta format in the input box.
5. Set the parameters default except Database option to PDB and click search button.
6. As soon as the search process completes the results are displayed
7. BLAST output includes the graphical overview box, a matching list and a text description of the alignment.

Result:

The similarity search for Ribokinase was performed.

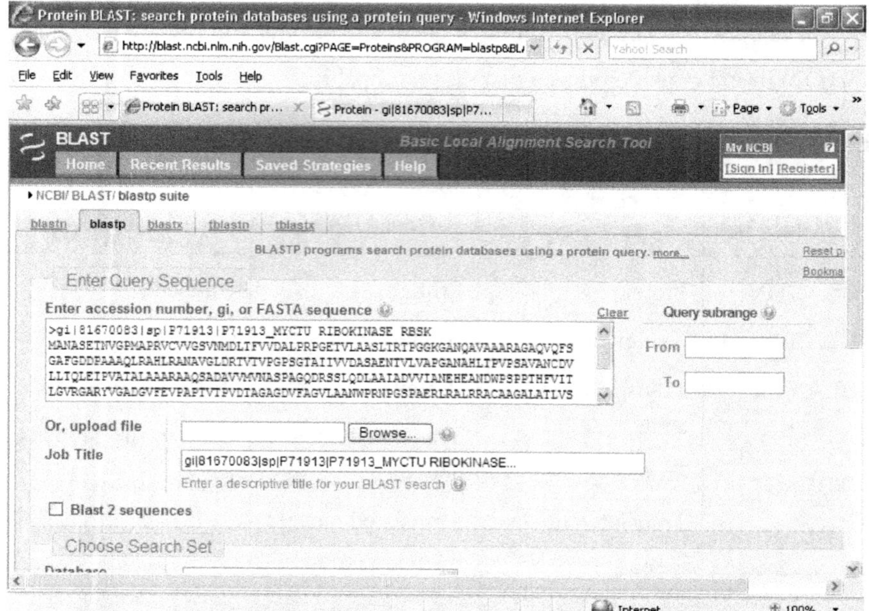

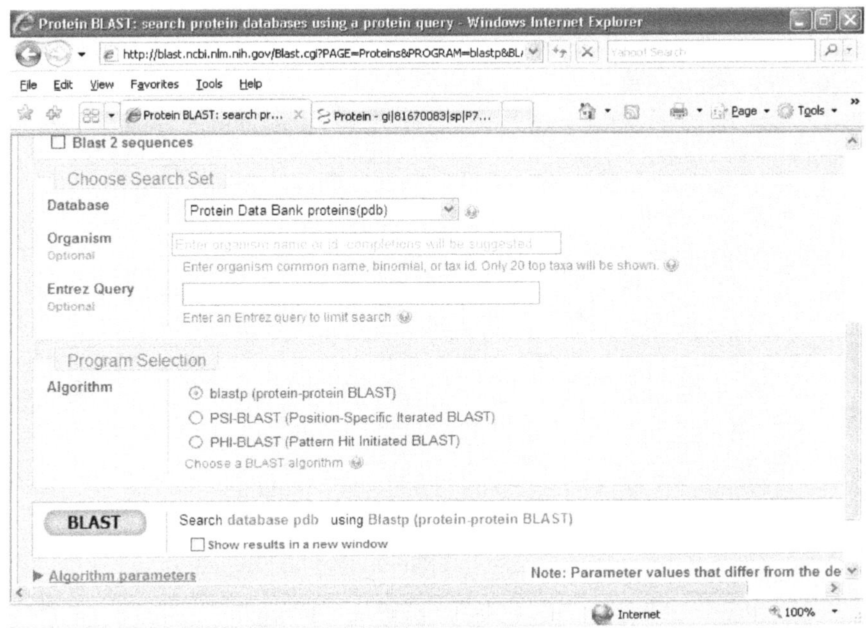

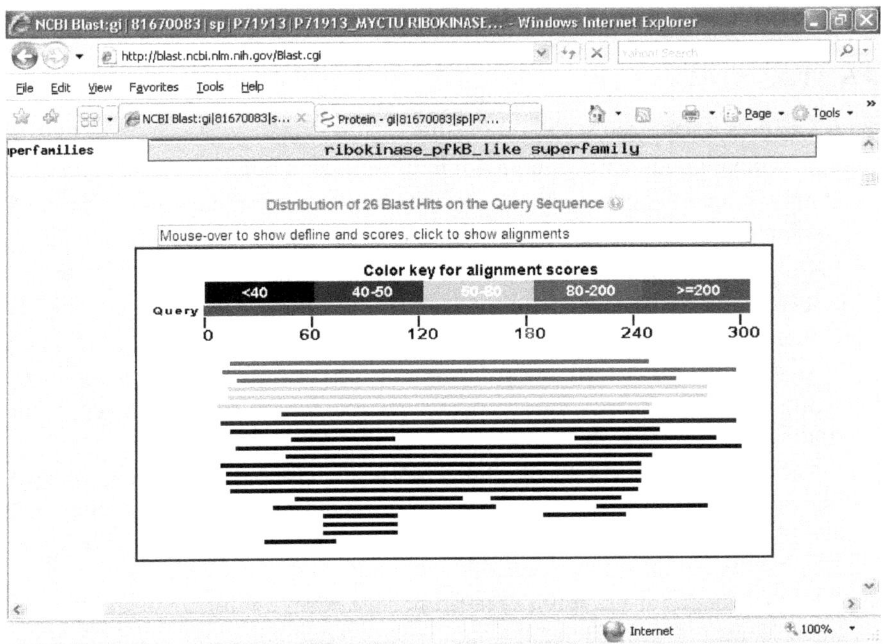

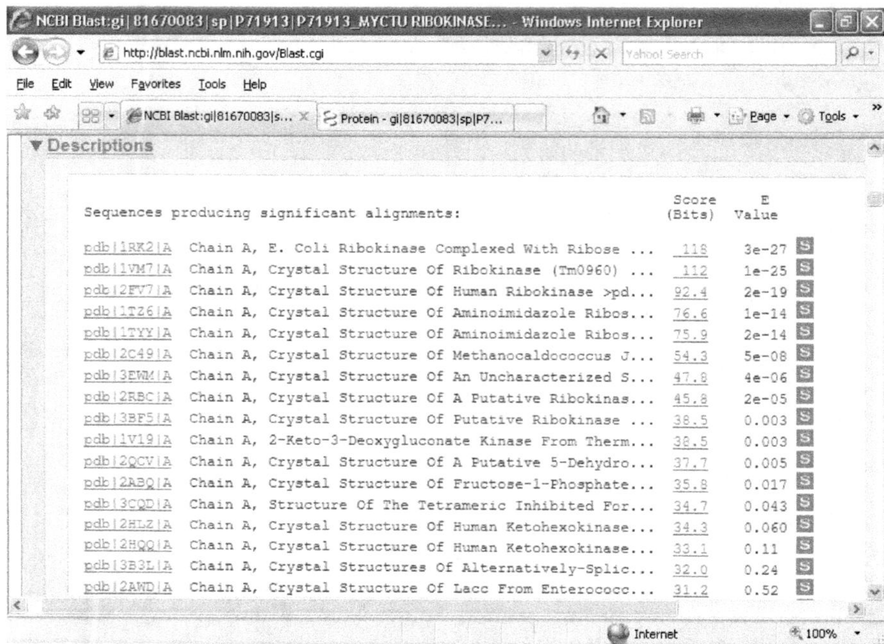

SIMILARITY SEARCH TOOLS- FASTA

FASTA

- ➢ FASTA is a database search algorithm
- ➢ It was developed at Virginia institute of bioinformatics
- ➢ It uses Pearson and lipman algorithm to search for similarities between of the same type as the query sequence.
- ➢ FASTA is a word based method. It looks for matching 'word' or the sequence patterns called k-tuples.
- ➢ It then builds a local alignment based upon the word matches
- ➢ It makes a list of all the words in each sequence. It matches identical words from each list and then creates diagonals by goining adjacent matches.
- ➢ FASTA then rescores the highest scoring regions using a replacement matrix (ex: PAM, BLOSUM).the best of these scores is called init 1.FASTA joins together the high scoring diagonals allowing for gaps. The best score from that is called initn
- ➢ FASTA finally uses smith-waterman algorithm to identify an optimal local alignment around the regions it has discovered.

IMPLEMENTATIONS OF FASTA

- ➢ *FASTA:* It compares a protein sequence to another protein sequence or a protein library or a DNA sequence to another DNA sequence.

- ➢ *TFASTA:* It compares a protein sequence to a DNA sequence by translating the DNA sequence in all 6possiblereading frames and then comparing each frame to a protein sequence.

- ➢ *LFASTA:* It identifies one or more regions of similaritybetween two sequences.

- ➢ *PLFASTA:* It presents a dot matrix plot of regions of sequence similarity between two sequences.

- ➢ *FASTX AND FASTY:* To translate probe DNA sequence in 3 reading frames and compare all the 3 frames to a protein sequence database.

FASTA FORMAT

- ➢ FASTA is one of the simplest and most popular sequence format, since it contains protein sequence information that is easily readable the analysis programs.

- ➢ It has a single definition line that begins with right handed bracket followed by a sequence name.

- ➢ The plane sequence in standard one retrieval symbols starts in the second line. Each line of the sequence data is limited to 60-80characters in width.

Statistical significance of FASTA

FASTA also uses E-values and bit scores and the estimation of these parameters in FASTA is essentially the same as in BLAST. However, FASTA output provides one more statistical parameters called z-score. This describes the number of standard deviations from the mean score for the database search.

Z score>15 → extremely significant match

Z 5-15 → highly probable homologs

Z<5 → distant relationship

Higher the z-score reported, more significant is the match.

Exercise: 8

Aim: To perform FASTA for the following sequence.

```
>tr|P71913|P71913_MYCTU RIBOKINASE RBSK

MANASETNVGPMAPRVCVVGSVNMDLTFVVDALPRPGETVLAASLTRTPGGKGANQAVAA
ARAGAQVQFSGAFGDDPAAAQLRAHLRANAVGLDRTVTVPGPSGTAIIVVDASAENTVLV
```

Procedure

1. The Ribokinase protein of mycobacterium tuberculosis sequence (P71913)was selected from the database.
2. login to http://www.ebi.ac.uk/Tools/fasta33/index.html
3. Paste the protein sequence in fasta format in the input box.
4. Set the parameters default and click RUN button.
5. As soon as the search process completes the results are displayed
6. FASTA output includes a matching list and a text description of the sequences which has shown the similarity.
7. By clicking show alignment button it displays the alignment of query protein to that of the similarity sequences.

Result

The similarity search for Ribokinase was performed using FASTA.

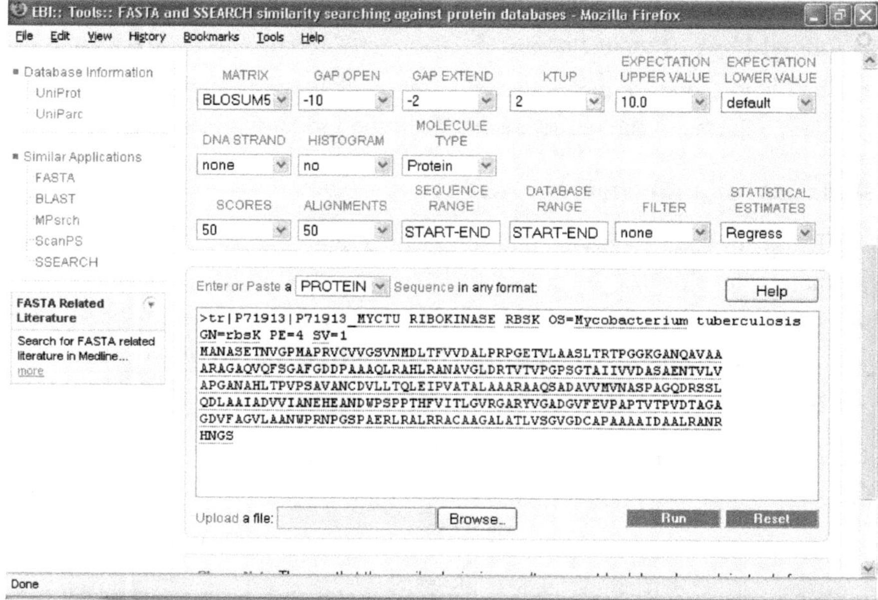

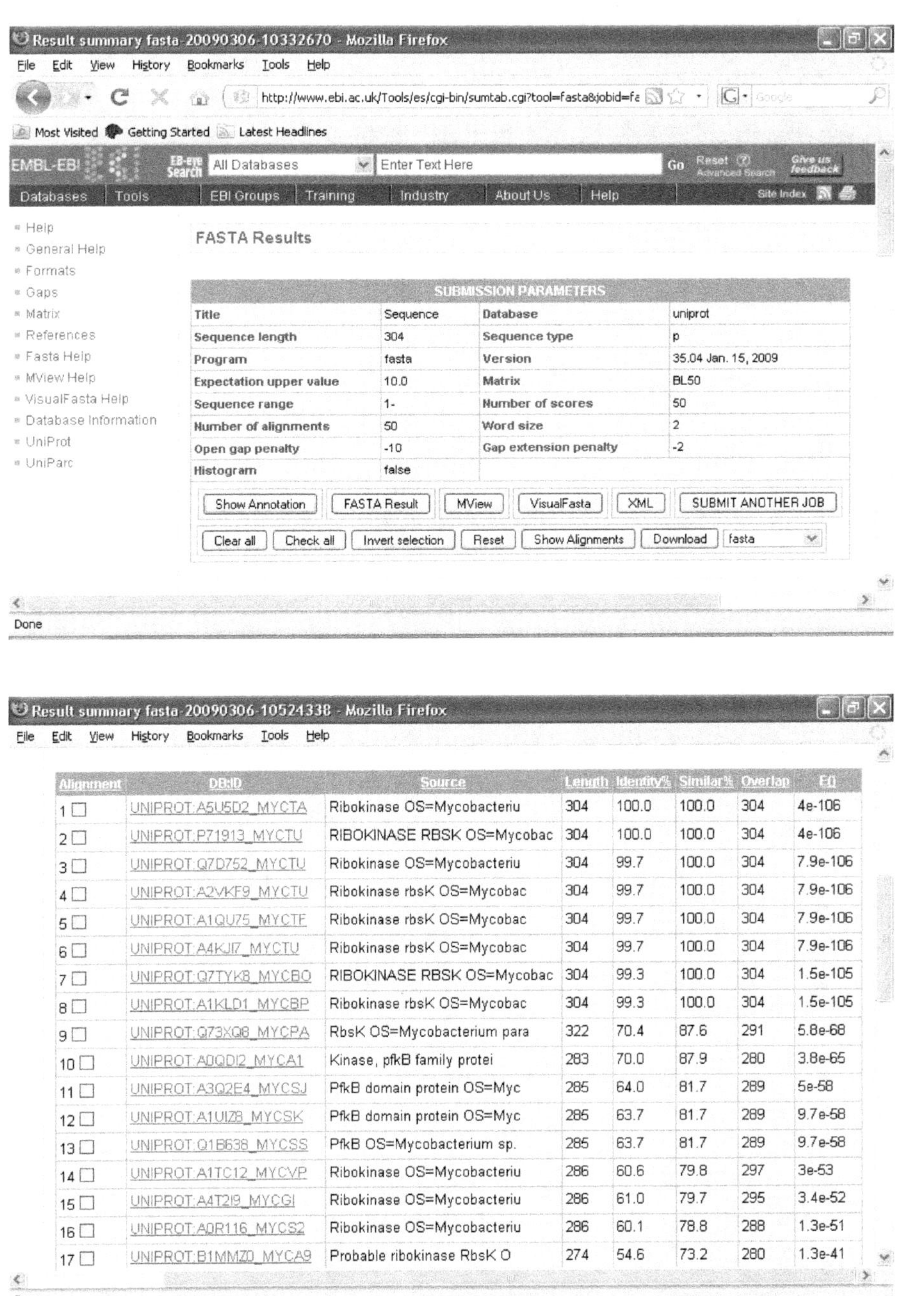

Alignment	DB:ID	Source	Length	Identity%	Similar%	Overlap	E()
1 ☐	UNIPROT:A5U5D2_MYCTA	Ribokinase OS=Mycobacteriu	304	100.0	100.0	304	4e-106
2 ☐	UNIPROT:P71913_MYCTU	RIBOKINASE RBSK OS=Mycobac	304	100.0	100.0	304	4e-106
3 ☐	UNIPROT:Q7D752_MYCTU	Ribokinase OS=Mycobacteriu	304	99.7	100.0	304	7.9e-106
4 ☐	UNIPROT:A2VKF9_MYCTU	Ribokinase rbsK OS=Mycobac	304	99.7	100.0	304	7.9e-106
5 ☐	UNIPROT:A1QU75_MYCTF	Ribokinase rbsK OS=Mycobac	304	99.7	100.0	304	7.9e-106
6 ☐	UNIPROT:A4KJI7_MYCTU	Ribokinase rbsK OS=Mycobac	304	99.7	100.0	304	7.9e-106
7 ☐	UNIPROT:Q7TYK8_MYCBO	RIBOKINASE RBSK OS=Mycobac	304	99.3	100.0	304	1.5e-105
8 ☐	UNIPROT:A1KLD1_MYCBP	Ribokinase rbsK OS=Mycobac	304	99.3	100.0	304	1.5e-105
9 ☐	UNIPROT:Q73XQ8_MYCPA	RbsK OS=Mycobacterium para	322	70.4	87.6	291	5.8e-68
10 ☐	UNIPROT:A0QDI2_MYCA1	Kinase, pfkB family protei	283	70.0	87.9	280	3.8e-65
11 ☐	UNIPROT:A3Q2E4_MYCSJ	PfkB domain protein OS=Myc	285	64.0	81.7	289	5e-58
12 ☐	UNIPROT:A1UIZ8_MYCSK	PfkB domain protein OS=Myc	285	63.7	81.7	289	9.7e-58
13 ☐	UNIPROT:Q1B638_MYCSS	PfkB OS=Mycobacterium sp.	285	63.7	81.7	289	9.7e-58
14 ☐	UNIPROT:A1TC12_MYCVP	Ribokinase OS=Mycobacteriu	286	60.6	79.8	297	3e-53
15 ☐	UNIPROT:A4T2I9_MYCGI	Ribokinase OS=Mycobacteriu	286	61.0	79.7	295	3.4e-52
16 ☐	UNIPROT:A0R116_MYCS2	Ribokinase OS=Mycobacteriu	286	60.1	78.8	288	1.3e-51
17 ☐	UNIPROT:B1MMZ0_MYCA9	Probable ribokinase RbsK O	274	54.6	73.2	280	1.3e-41

Result summary fasta-20090306-10524338 - Mozilla Firefox

File Edit View History Bookmarks Tools Help

#		UNIPROT ID	Description					
18	☐	UNIPROT:Q0SH59_RHOSR	Ribokinase OS=Rhodococcus	288	49.0	70.1	294	9.5e-36
19	☐	UNIPROT:Q5Z026_NOCFA	Putative ribokinase OS=Noc	287	46.9	68.5	292	3.5e-33
20	☐	UNIPROT:A5CPI2_CLAM3	Putative ribokinase OS=Cla	276	43.3	68.2	289	9.7e-25
21	☐	UNIPROT:A3TQ35_9MICO	Ribokinase OS=Janibacter s	276	42.3	65.1	281	4.9e-24
22	☐	UNIPROT:B0RAF6_CLAMS	Carbohydrate kinase OS=Cla	270	42.4	66.4	283	1.2e-23
23	☐	UNIPROT:A8M5C8_SALAI	PfkB domain protein OS=Sal	296	43.0	67.9	293	1.5e-22
24	☐	UNIPROT:B4W8B9_9CAUL	Kinase, pfkB family OS=Bre	282	38.6	65.2	293	2.8e-22
25	☐	UNIPROT:A4X472_SALTO	PfkB domain protein OS=Sal	298	43.1	67.6	299	1.7e-21
26	☐	UNIPROT:Q5KUX1_GEOKA	Ribokinase OS=Geobacillus	297	35.8	61.9	302	3.2e-21
27	☐	UNIPROT:Q0C5Q3_HYPNA	Ribokinase OS=Hyphomonas n	280	38.3	63.1	290	3.5e-21
28	☐	UNIPROT:A8VYI9_9BACI	FAD dependent oxidoreducta	292	35.8	62.2	296	4.2e-21
29	☐	UNIPROT:A5UYD8_ROSS1	Ribokinase OS=Roseiflexus	305	40.5	64.0	311	6.5e-21
30	☐	UNIPROT:B4BQZ6_9BACI	Ribokinase OS=Geobacillus	298	35.8	60.9	302	1.4e-20
31	☐	UNIPROT:Q3IYI7_RHOS4	Putative RbsK, Carbohydrat	284	38.3	62.4	290	3.5e-20
32	☐	UNIPROT:B7YAS9_9BACI	Ribokinase OS=Geobacillus	297	35.8	60.9	302	4.2e-20
33	☐	UNIPROT:Q9RZ99_DEIRA	Ribokinase OS=Deinococcus	300	44.6	62.4	303	4.8e-20
34	☐	UNIPROT:A3PNR3_RHOS1	PfkB domain protein OS=Rho	284	39.4	60.6	292	5.3e-20
35	☐	UNIPROT:RBSK_BACHD	Ribokinase OS=Bacillus halod	294	35.4	61.3	297	1.1e-19
36	☐	UNIPROT:A7BBS3_9ACTO	Putative uncharacterized p	301	39.4	63.9	310	1.1e-19

Done

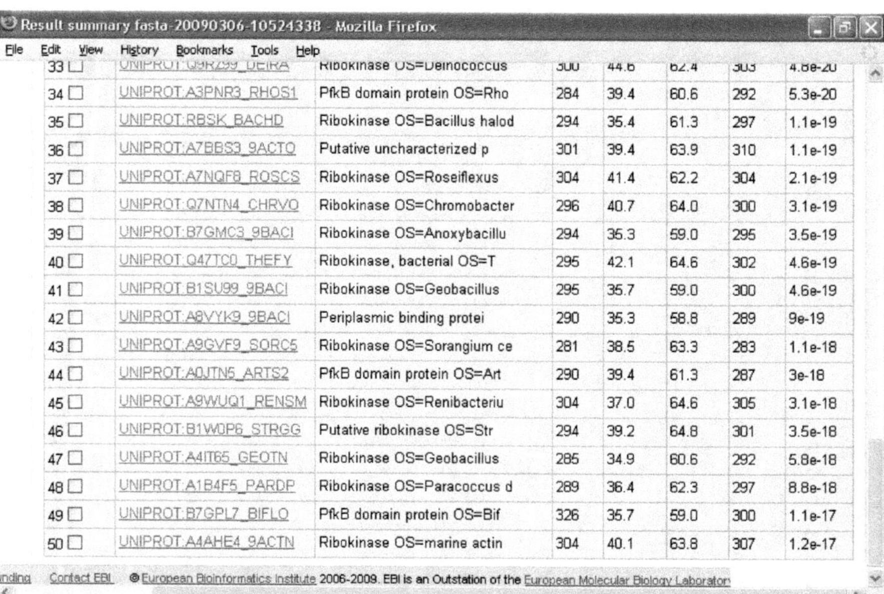

Result summary fasta-20090306-10524338 - Mozilla Firefox

File Edit View History Bookmarks Tools Help

#		UNIPROT ID	Description					
33	☐	UNIPROT:Q9RZ99_DEIRA	Ribokinase OS=Deinococcus	300	44.6	62.4	303	4.8e-20
34	☐	UNIPROT:A3PNR3_RHOS1	PfkB domain protein OS=Rho	284	39.4	60.6	292	5.3e-20
35	☐	UNIPROT:RBSK_BACHD	Ribokinase OS=Bacillus halod	294	35.4	61.3	297	1.1e-19
36	☐	UNIPROT:A7BBS3_9ACTO	Putative uncharacterized p	301	39.4	63.9	310	1.1e-19
37	☐	UNIPROT:A7NQF8_ROSCS	Ribokinase OS=Roseiflexus	304	41.4	62.2	304	2.1e-19
38	☐	UNIPROT:Q7NTN4_CHRVO	Ribokinase OS=Chromobacter	296	40.7	64.0	300	3.1e-19
39	☐	UNIPROT:B7GMC3_9BACI	Ribokinase OS=Anoxybacillu	294	35.3	59.0	295	3.5e-19
40	☐	UNIPROT:Q47TC0_THEFY	Ribokinase, bacterial OS=T	295	42.1	64.6	302	4.6e-19
41	☐	UNIPROT:B1SU99_9BACI	Ribokinase OS=Geobacillus	295	35.7	59.0	300	4.6e-19
42	☐	UNIPROT:A8VYK9_9BACI	Periplasmic binding protei	290	35.3	58.8	289	9e-19
43	☐	UNIPROT:A9GVF9_SORC5	Ribokinase OS=Sorangium ce	281	38.5	63.3	283	1.1e-18
44	☐	UNIPROT:A0JTN5_ARTS2	PfkB domain protein OS=Art	290	39.4	61.3	287	3e-18
45	☐	UNIPROT:A9WUQ1_RENSM	Ribokinase OS=Renibacteriu	304	37.0	64.6	305	3.1e-18
46	☐	UNIPROT:B1W0P6_STRGG	Putative ribokinase OS=Str	294	39.2	64.8	301	3.5e-18
47	☐	UNIPROT:A4IT65_GEOTN	Ribokinase OS=Geobacillus	285	34.9	60.6	292	5.8e-18
48	☐	UNIPROT:A1B4F5_PARDP	Ribokinase OS=Paracoccus d	289	36.4	62.3	297	8.8e-18
49	☐	UNIPROT:B7GPL7_BIFLO	PfkB domain protein OS=Bif	326	35.7	59.0	300	1.1e-17
50	☐	UNIPROT:A4AHE4_9ACTN	Ribokinase OS=marine actin	304	40.1	63.8	307	1.2e-17

Done

3

Nucleic Acid Feature Identification

NUCLEIC ACID FEATURES PREDICTION

Deoxyribonucleic acid is a double stranded genetic material present in most of the organisms. This genomic DNA differs from prokaryotes to eukaryotes.

GENOMIC DNA FEATURES OF PROKARYOTES

Prokaryotes include bacteria, archaea; eukarya that have relatively small genomes with sizes ranging from 0.5to10mbp.The gene density in these genomes is very high; since very few repetitive sequences are present.

In bacteria, majority of genes have a start codon ATG which codes for methionine.The other codons like GTG and TTG along with ATG form the initiation codons which starts the process of translation. To identify this initiation codon, a sequence called shine dalgarno sequence which is a stretch of purine rich sequence complementary to 16s rRNA in the ribosome tail. At the end there is a stop codon and poly T tail is present. Any prokaryotic genes are transferred together as one operon.

GENOMIC DNA FEATURES IN EUKARYOTES

These genomes are much larger than prokaryotic ones. Its sizes ranging from 10mbp to 670gbp. They tend to have very low gene density. Since the space between genes is often very large and rich, repetitive sequences occur. Most importantly genomic DNA is characterized by mosaic organization in which a gene is split into pieces called 'exons' by intervening non-coding sequences called 'introns'.

The nascent transcript from a eukaryotic gene is modified in 3 different ways, before undergoing translation which include 5' capping, splicing and 3` poly adenylation. These genomes consist of kozak sequences as a start codon and poly A tail at the termination, which locate the final coding sequence. The splice site consists of GTAACT as a consensus motif since the splice section of introns & exons following GT-AG rules for splicing. The CG island is a short stretch of DNA in which the frequency of the CG sequence is higher than other regions. It is also called the CpG island, where "p" simply indicates that "C" and "G" are connected by a phosphodiester bond.The HMM can be used to find if a given short sequence, the sequence comes from CpG islands or not. The HMM can also be trained to find the CpG islands in a long sequence.

CpG islands are often located around the promoters of **housekeeping genes** (which are essential for general cell functions) or other genes frequently expressed in a cell. At these locations, the CG sequence is not methylated. By contrast, the CG sequences in inactive genes are usually methylated to suppress their expression. Methylation of promoter-associated CGIs plays an important role in gene regulation and carcinogenesis. Because of the functional importance, multiple algorithms have been available for identifying CGIs in a sequence.

Functional units of DNA (Genes) can be identified by different gene-finding programs, such as GeneMark, GlimmerM, GRAIL, GenScan, and Fgenes.RepeatMasker is a program that screens DNA sequences for interspersed repeats and low complexity DNA sequences.

FEATURES OF GENOMIC DNA SEQUENCE

Introduction

Deoxyribonucleic acid is a double standard genetic material present in most of the organisms. This genomic DNA differs from prokaryotes to eukaryotes.

Genomic DNA Features of Prokaryotes

Prokaryotes include bacteria, archaea; eukarya that have relatively small genomes with sizes ranging from 0.5to10mbp.The gene density in these genomes is very high; since very few repetitive sequences are present.

In bacteria, majority of genes have a start codon ATG which codes for methionine.The other codons like GTG and TTG along with ATG form the initiation codons which starts the process of translation. To identify this initiation codon, a sequence called shine dalgarno sequence, is a stretch of purine rich sequence complementary to 16s rRNA in the ribosome tail. At the end there is a stop codon and poly T tail is present. Any prokaryotic genes are transferred together as one operon.

Genomic DNA Features in Eukaryotes

These genomes are much larger than prokaryotic ones. It's sizes ranging from 10mbp to 670gbp.They tend to have very low gene density. Since the space between genes is often very large and rich, repetitive sequences occur. Most importantly genomic DNA is characterized by mosaic organization, in which a gene is split in to pieces called 'exons' by intervening non-coding sequences called 'introns'.

The nascent transcript from a eukaryotic gene is modified in 3 different ways, before undergoing translation which include 5' capping, splicing and 3` poly adenylation. These genomes consist of kozak sequences as a start codon and poly A tail at the termination, locate the final coding sequence. The splice site consists of GTAACT as a consensus motif since the splice section of introns &exons following GT-AG rules for splicing.CG Islands are the regions in DNA sequences where the dimer CG repeatedly occurs. The HMM can be used to find if a given short sequence, the sequence comes form CpG islands or not. The HMM can also be trained to find the CpG islands in a long sequence.

Exercise: 9

GenScan

Aim: To predict the exon and intron regions of the given DNA sequence (*Homo sapiens* leptin – lep, 3444 bp, NM_000230)

Procedure

- Retrieve the query DNA sequence in FASTA format by accessing the nucleotide database.
- Login into http://genes.mit.edu/GENSCAN.html and paste the sequence in input box.
- Click run button.
- As soon as the run button is clicked the process continues for predicting the gene structure.
- The results are obtained after the analysis.

Result

Two Exons have been predicted from regions 58 to 561 and 1650 to 1655.

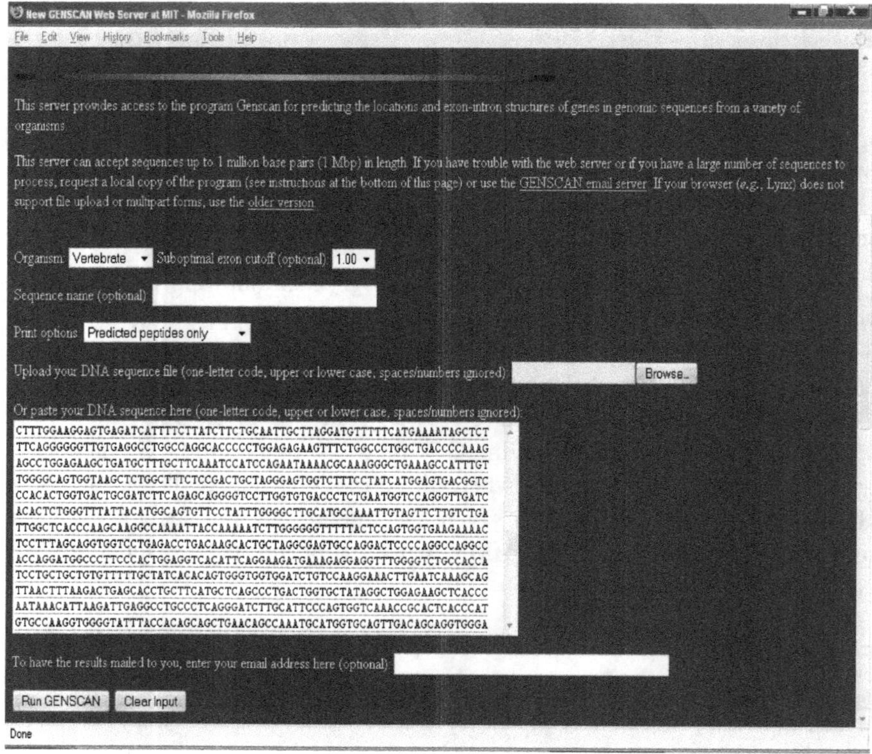
New GENSCAN Web Server at MIT - Mozilla Firefox
File Edit View History Bookmarks Tools Help
This server provides access to the program Genscan for predicting the locations and exon-intron structures of genes in genomic sequences from a variety of organisms.
This server can accept sequences up to 1 million base pairs (1 Mbp) in length. If you have trouble with the web server or if you have a large number of sequences to process, request a local copy of the program (see instructions at the bottom of this page) or use the GENSCAN email server. If your browser (e.g., Lynx) does not support file upload or multipart forms, use the older version.
Organism: Vertebrate   Suboptimal exon cutoff (optional): 1.00
Sequence name (optional):
Print options: Predicted peptides only
Upload your DNA sequence file (one-letter code, upper or lower case, spaces/numbers ignored)   Browse...
Or paste your DNA sequence here (one-letter code, upper or lower case, spaces/numbers ignored):
CTTTGGAAGGAGTGAGATCATTTTCTTATCTTCTGCAATTGCTTAGGATGTTTTTCATGAAAATAGCTCT
TTCAGGGGGGTTGTGAGGCCTGGCCAGGCACCCCCTGGAGAGAAGTTTCTGGCCCTGGCTGACCCCAAAG
AGCCTGGAGAAGCTGATGCTTTGCTTCAAATCCATCCAGAATAAAACGCAAAGGGCTGAAAGCCATTTGT
TGGGGCAGTGGTAAGCTCTGGCTTTCTCCGACTGCTAGGGAGTGGTCTTTCCTATCATGGAGTGACGGTC
CCACACTGGTGACTGCGATCTTCAGAGCAGGGGTCCTTGGTGTGACCCTCTGAATGGTCCAGGGTTGATC
ACACTCTGGGTTTATTACATGGCAGTGTTCCTATTTGGGGCTTGCATGCCAAATTGTAGTTCTTGTCTGA
TTGGCTCACCCAAGCAAGGCCAAAATTACCAAAAATCTTGGGGGGTTTTTACTCCAGTGGTGAAGAAAAC
TCCTTTAGCAGGTGGTCCTGAGACCTGACAAGCACTGCTAGGCGAGTGCCAGGACTCCCCAGGCCAGGCC
ACCAGGATGGCCCTTCCCACTGGAGGTCACATTCAGGAAGATGAAAGAGGAGGTTTGGGGTCTGCCACCA
TCCTGCTGCTGTGTTTTTGCTATCACACAGTGGGTGGTGGATCTGTCCAAGGAAACTTGAATCAAAGCAG
TTAACTTTAAGACTGAGCACCTGCTTCATGCTCAGCCCTGACTGGTGCTATAGGCTGGAGAAGCTCACCC
AATAAACATTAAGATTGAGGCCTGCCCTCAGGGATCTTGCATTCCCAGTGGTCAAACCGCACTCACCCAT
GTGCCAAGGTGGGGTATTTACCACAGCAGCTGAACAGCCAAATGCATGGTGCAGTTGACAGCAGGTGGGA
To have the results mailed to you, enter your email address here (optional):
Run GENSCAN   Clear Input
Done

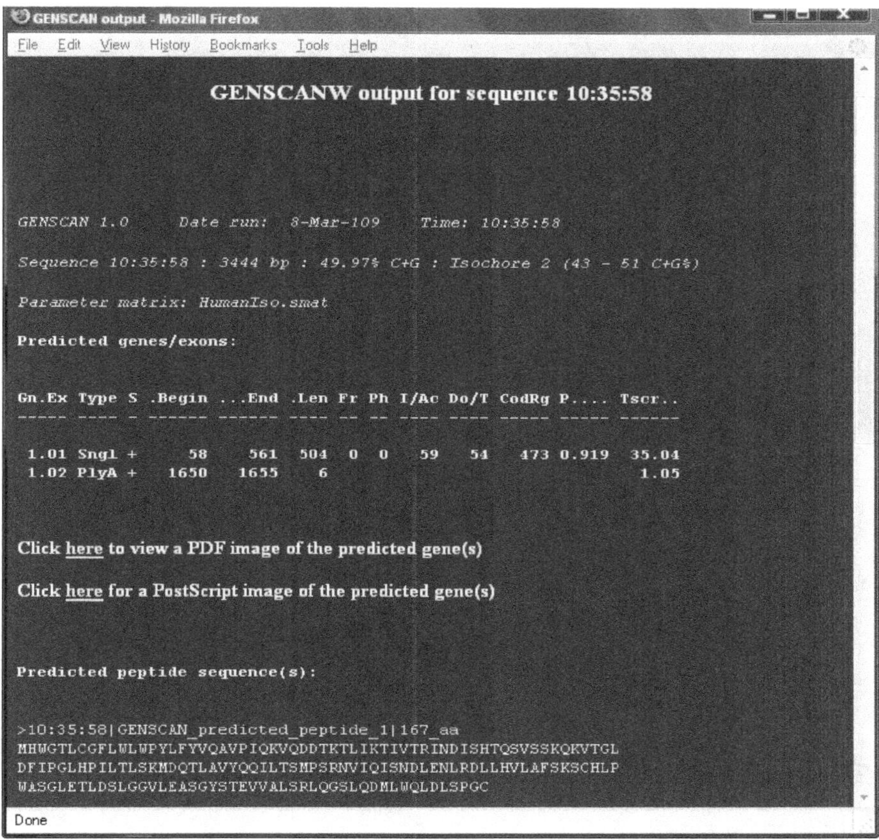
GENSCAN output - Mozilla Firefox
File   Edit   View   History   Bookmarks   Tools   Help

GENSCANW output for sequence 10:35:58

GENSCAN 1.0   Date run: 8-Mar-109   Time: 10:35:58

Sequence 10:35:58 : 3444 bp : 49.97% C+G : Isochore 2 (43 - 51 C+G%)

Parameter matrix: HumanIso.smat

Predicted genes/exons:

Gn.Ex Type S .Begin ...End .Len Fr Ph I/Ac Do/T CodRg P.... Tscr..
----- ---- - ------ ------ ---- -- -- ---- ---- ----- ----- ------

 1.01 Sngl +   58   561 504 0 0   59   54   473 0.919 35.04
 1.02 PlyA +   1650   1655   6   1.05

Click here to view a PDF image of the predicted gene(s)

Click here for a PostScript image of the predicted gene(s)

Predicted peptide sequence(s):

>10:35:58|GENSCAN_predicted_peptide_1|167_aa
MHWGTLCGFLWLWPYLFYVQAVPIQKVQDDTKTLIKTIVTRINDISHTQSVSSKQKVTGL
DFIPGLHPILTLSKMDQTLAVYQQILTSMPSRNVIQISNDLENLRDLLHVLAFSKSCHLP
WASGLETLDSLGGVLEASGYSTEVVALSRLQGSLQDMLWQLDLSPGC

Done

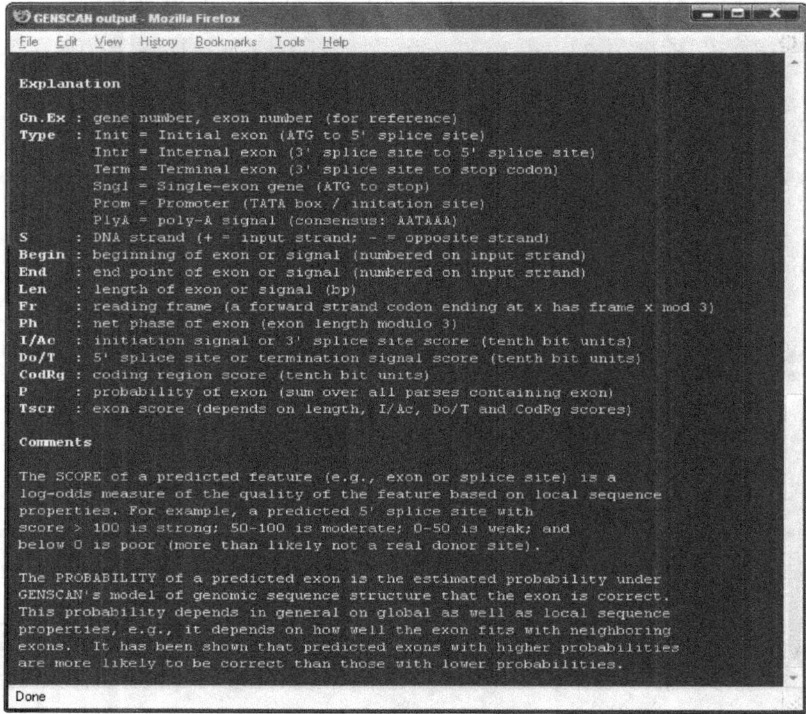

Exercise: 10

Splice Predictor

Aim: To predict the splice sites of the given DNA sequence (*Homo sapiens* leptin – lep, 3444 bp, NM_000230)

Procedure

- Retrieve the query DNA sequence in FASTA format by accessing the nucleotide database.
- Login to http://deepc2.psi.iastate.edu/cgi-bin/sp.cgi and paste the sequence in input box.
- Click run button.
- As soon as the run button is clicked the process continues for predicting the gene structure.
- The results are obtained after the analysis.

Result

16 splice sites have been predicted.

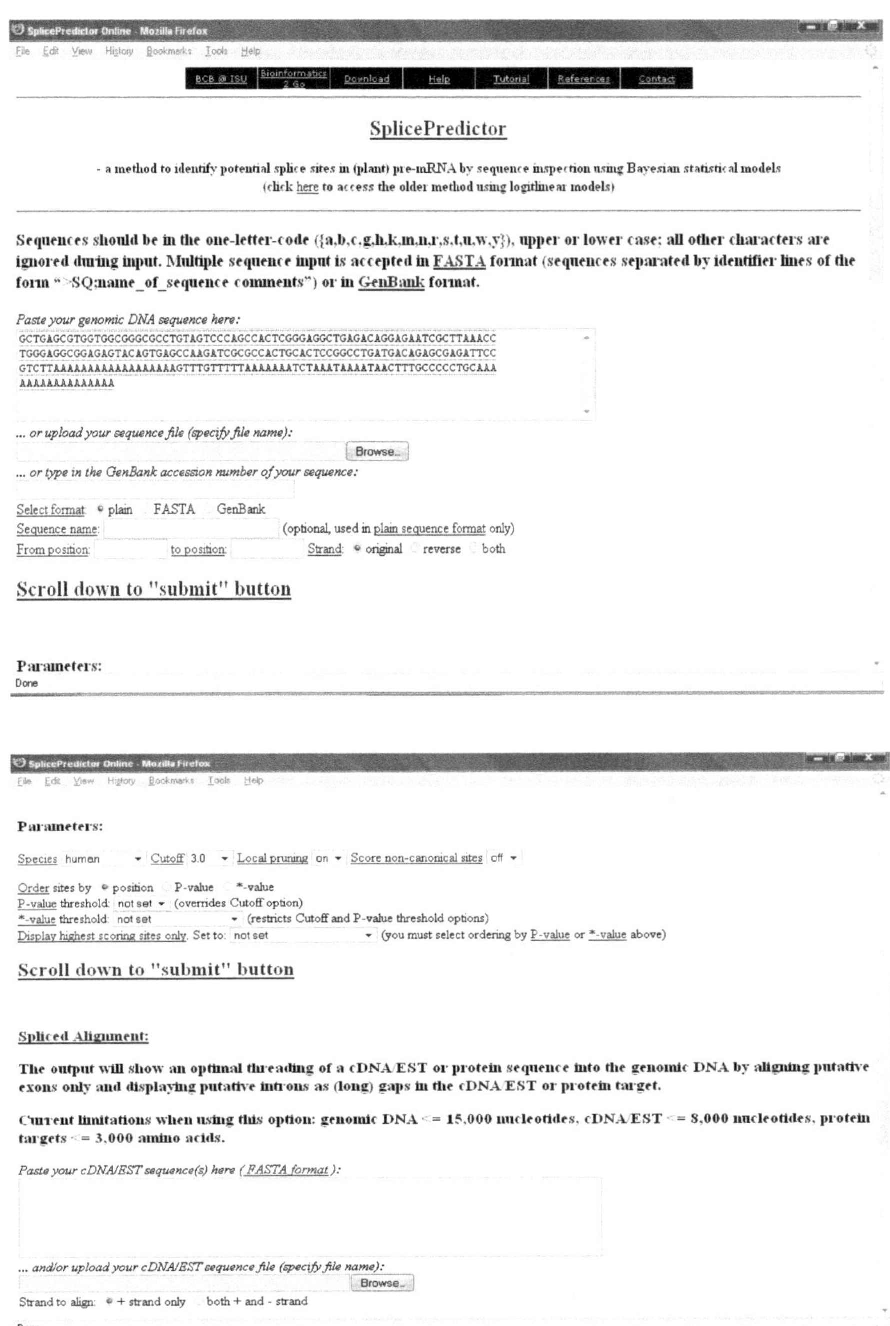

SplicePredictor Online - Mozilla Firefox
File Edit View History Bookmarks Tools Help
BCB @ ISU | Bioinformatics 2 Go | Download | Help | Tutorial | References | Contact

SplicePredictor

- a method to identify potential splice sites in (plant) pre-mRNA by sequence inspection using Bayesian statistical models
(click here to access the older method using logitlinear models)

Sequences should be in the one-letter-code ({a,b,c,g,h,k,m,n,r,s,t,u,w,y}), upper or lower case; all other characters are ignored during input. Multiple sequence input is accepted in FASTA format (sequences separated by identifier lines of the form ">SQ:name_of_sequence comments") or in GenBank format.

Paste your genomic DNA sequence here:
GCTGAGCGTGGTGGCGGGCGCCTGTAGTCCCAGCCACTCGGGAGGCTGAGACAGGAGAATCGCTTAAACC
TGGGAGGCGGAGAGTACAGTGAGCCAAGATCGCGCCACTGCACTCCGGCCTGATGACAGAGCGAGATTCC
GTCTTAAAAAAAAAAAAAAAAAAAAGTTTGTTTTTAAAAAAATCTAAATAAAATAACTTTGCCCCCTGCAAA
AAAAAAAAAAAAAA

... or upload your sequence file (specify file name):
[Browse...]
... or type in the GenBank accession number of your sequence:

Select format: ● plain   FASTA   GenBank
Sequence name: (optional, used in plain sequence format only)
From position: to position: Strand: ● original   reverse   both

Scroll down to "submit" button

Parameters:
Done

SplicePredictor Online - Mozilla Firefox
File Edit View History Bookmarks Tools Help

Parameters:

Species human   ▼   Cutoff 3.0   ▼ Local pruning on ▼ Score non-canonical sites off ▼

Order sites by ● position   P-value   *-value
P-value threshold: not set ▼ (overrides Cutoff option)
*-value threshold: not set   ▼ (restricts Cutoff and P-value threshold options)
Display highest scoring sites only. Set to: not set   ▼ (you must select ordering by P-value or *-value above)

Scroll down to "submit" button

Spliced Alignment:

The output will show an optimal threading of a cDNA/EST or protein sequence into the genomic DNA by aligning putative exons only and displaying putative introns as (long) gaps in the cDNA/EST or protein target.

Current limitations when using this option: genomic DNA <= 15,000 nucleotides, cDNA/EST <= 8,000 nucleotides, protein targets <= 3,000 amino acids.

Paste your cDNA/EST sequence(s) here (FASTA format):

... and/or upload your cDNA/EST sequence file (specify file name):
[Browse...]
Strand to align: ● + strand only   both + and - strand
Done

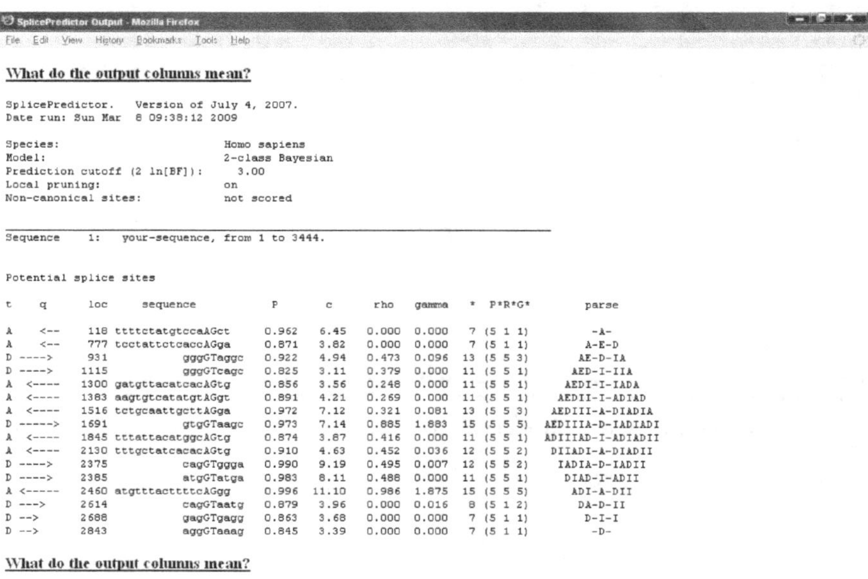

Output:

```
SplicePredictor.    Version of July 4, 2007.
Date run: Sun Mar  8 09:38:12 2009

Species:                 Homo sapiens
Model:                   2-class Bayesian
Prediction cutoff (2 ln[BF]):    3.00
Local pruning:           on
Non-canonical sites:     not scored


Sequence    1:    your-sequence, from 1 to 3444.


Potential splice sites

t      q       loc     sequence         P      c      rho    gamma   *  P*R*G*        parse

A      <--     118 ttttctatgtccaAGct    0.962  6.45   0.000  0.000   7 (5 1 1)          -A-
A      <--     777 tcctattctcaccAGga    0.871  3.82   0.000  0.000   7 (5 1 1)         A-E-D
D ---->        931         gggGTaggc    0.922  4.94   0.473  0.096  13 (5 5 3)         AE-D-IA
D ---->        1115        gggGTcagc    0.825  3.11   0.379  0.000  11 (5 5 1)        AED-I-IIA
A <----        1300 gatgttacatcacAGtg    0.856  3.56   0.248  0.000  11 (5 5 1)       AEDI-I-IADA
A <----        1383 aagtgtcatatgtAGgt    0.891  4.21   0.269  0.000  11 (5 5 1)       AEDII-I-ADIAD
A <----        1516 tctgcaattgcttAGga    0.972  7.12   0.321  0.081  13 (5 5 3)      AEDIII-A-DIADIA
D ----->       1691        gtgGTaagc    0.973  7.14   0.885  1.883  15 (5 5 5)    AEDIIIA-D-IADIADI
A <----        1845 tttattacatggcAGtg    0.874  3.87   0.416  0.000  11 (5 5 1)   ADIIIAD-I-ADIADII
A <----        2130 tttgctatcacacAGtg    0.910  4.63   0.452  0.036  12 (5 5 2)    DIIADI-A-DIADII
D ---->        2375        cagGTggga    0.990  9.19   0.495  0.007  12 (5 5 2)     IADIA-D-IADII
D ---->        2385        atgGTatga    0.983  8.11   0.488  0.000  11 (5 5 1)      DIAD-I-ADII
A <-----       2460 atgtttacttttcAGgg    0.996 11.10   0.986  1.875  15 (5 5 5)       ADI-A-DII
D --->         2614        cagGTaatg    0.879  3.96   0.000  0.016   8 (5 1 2)        DA-D-II
D -->          2688        gagGTgagg    0.863  3.68   0.000  0.000   7 (5 1 1)         D-I-I
D -->          2843        aggGTaaag    0.845  3.39   0.000  0.000   7 (5 1 1)          -D-
```

What do the output columns mean?

Exercise: 11

CpG Islands

Aim: To predict the CpG Island regions of the given DNA sequence (*Homo sapiens* leptin – lep, 3444 bp, NM_000230)

Procedure

- Retrieve the query DNA sequence in FASTA format by accessing the nucleotide database.
- 12. Login to http://www.ualberta.ca/~stothard/javascript/cpg_islands.html and paste the sequence in input box.
- 13. Click run button.
- 14. As soon as the run button is clicked the process continues for predicting the gene structure.
- 15. The results are obtained after the analysis.

Result

CpG islands have been plotted at different places.

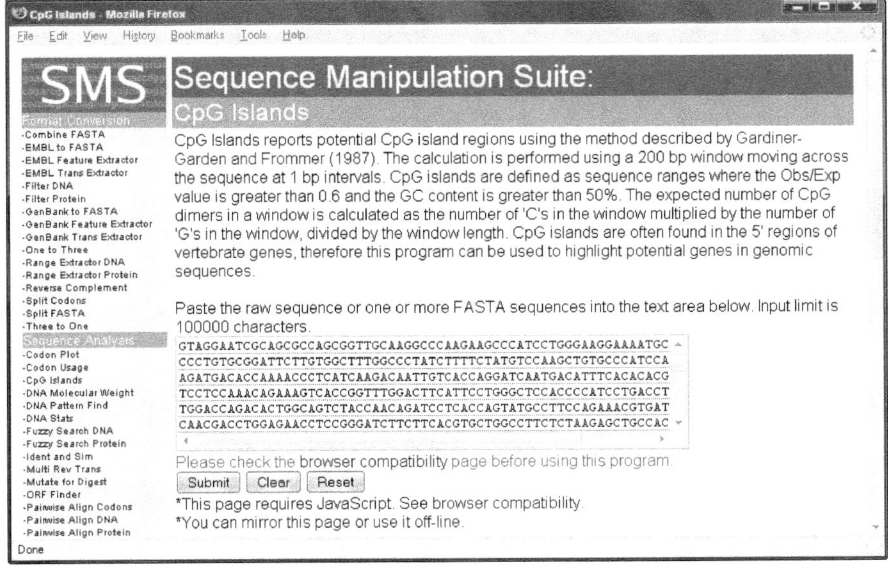

Output

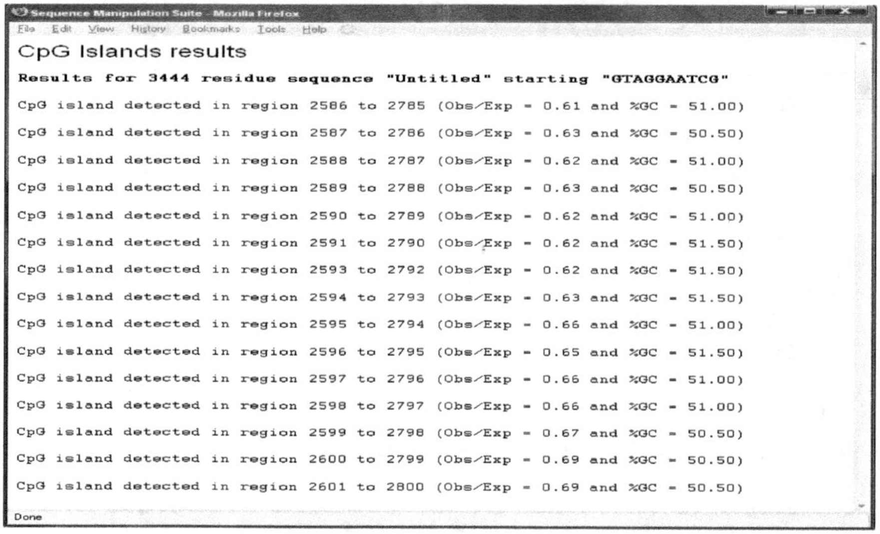

```
Sequence Manipulation Suite - Mozilla Firefox
File  Edit  View  History  Bookmarks  Tools  Help

CpG Islands results

Results for 3444 residue sequence "Untitled" starting "GTAGGAATCG"

CpG island detected in region 2586 to 2785 (Obs/Exp = 0.61 and %GC = 51.00)

CpG island detected in region 2587 to 2786 (Obs/Exp = 0.63 and %GC = 50.50)

CpG island detected in region 2588 to 2787 (Obs/Exp = 0.62 and %GC = 51.00)

CpG island detected in region 2589 to 2788 (Obs/Exp = 0.63 and %GC = 50.50)

CpG island detected in region 2590 to 2789 (Obs/Exp = 0.62 and %GC = 51.00)

CpG island detected in region 2591 to 2790 (Obs/Exp = 0.62 and %GC = 51.50)

CpG island detected in region 2593 to 2792 (Obs/Exp = 0.62 and %GC = 51.50)

CpG island detected in region 2594 to 2793 (Obs/Exp = 0.63 and %GC = 51.50)

CpG island detected in region 2595 to 2794 (Obs/Exp = 0.66 and %GC = 51.00)

CpG island detected in region 2596 to 2795 (Obs/Exp = 0.65 and %GC = 51.50)

CpG island detected in region 2597 to 2796 (Obs/Exp = 0.66 and %GC = 51.00)

CpG island detected in region 2598 to 2797 (Obs/Exp = 0.66 and %GC = 51.00)

CpG island detected in region 2599 to 2798 (Obs/Exp = 0.67 and %GC = 50.50)

CpG island detected in region 2600 to 2799 (Obs/Exp = 0.69 and %GC = 50.50)

CpG island detected in region 2601 to 2800 (Obs/Exp = 0.69 and %GC = 50.50)

Done
```

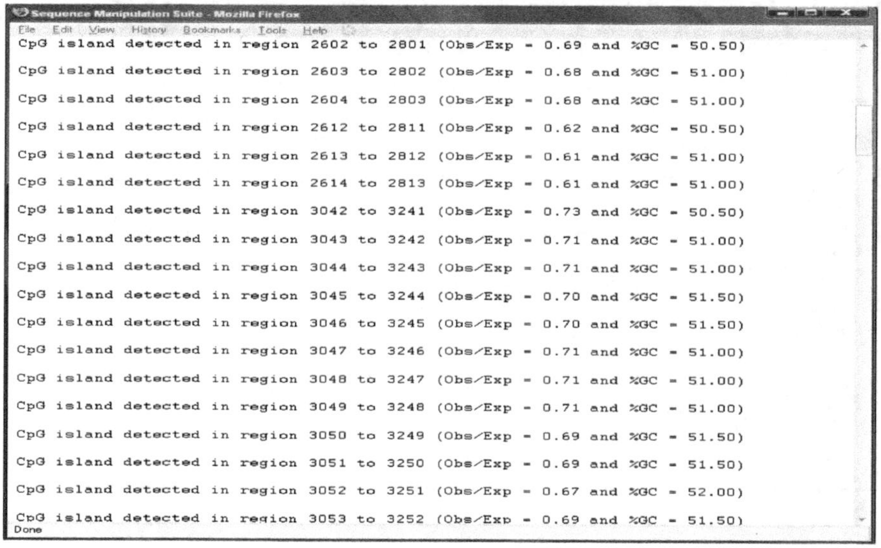

```
Sequence Manipulation Suite - Mozilla Firefox
File  Edit  View  History  Bookmarks  Tools  Help
CpG island detected in region 2602 to 2801 (Obs/Exp = 0.69 and %GC = 50.50)

CpG island detected in region 2603 to 2802 (Obs/Exp = 0.68 and %GC = 51.00)

CpG island detected in region 2604 to 2803 (Obs/Exp = 0.68 and %GC = 51.00)

CpG island detected in region 2612 to 2811 (Obs/Exp = 0.62 and %GC = 50.50)

CpG island detected in region 2613 to 2812 (Obs/Exp = 0.61 and %GC = 51.00)

CpG island detected in region 2614 to 2813 (Obs/Exp = 0.61 and %GC = 51.00)

CpG island detected in region 3042 to 3241 (Obs/Exp = 0.73 and %GC = 50.50)

CpG island detected in region 3043 to 3242 (Obs/Exp = 0.71 and %GC = 51.00)

CpG island detected in region 3044 to 3243 (Obs/Exp = 0.71 and %GC = 51.00)

CpG island detected in region 3045 to 3244 (Obs/Exp = 0.70 and %GC = 51.50)

CpG island detected in region 3046 to 3245 (Obs/Exp = 0.70 and %GC = 51.50)

CpG island detected in region 3047 to 3246 (Obs/Exp = 0.71 and %GC = 51.00)

CpG island detected in region 3048 to 3247 (Obs/Exp = 0.71 and %GC = 51.00)

CpG island detected in region 3049 to 3248 (Obs/Exp = 0.71 and %GC = 51.00)

CpG island detected in region 3050 to 3249 (Obs/Exp = 0.69 and %GC = 51.50)

CpG island detected in region 3051 to 3250 (Obs/Exp = 0.69 and %GC = 51.50)

CpG island detected in region 3052 to 3251 (Obs/Exp = 0.67 and %GC = 52.00)

CpG island detected in region 3053 to 3252 (Obs/Exp = 0.69 and %GC = 51.50)
Done
```

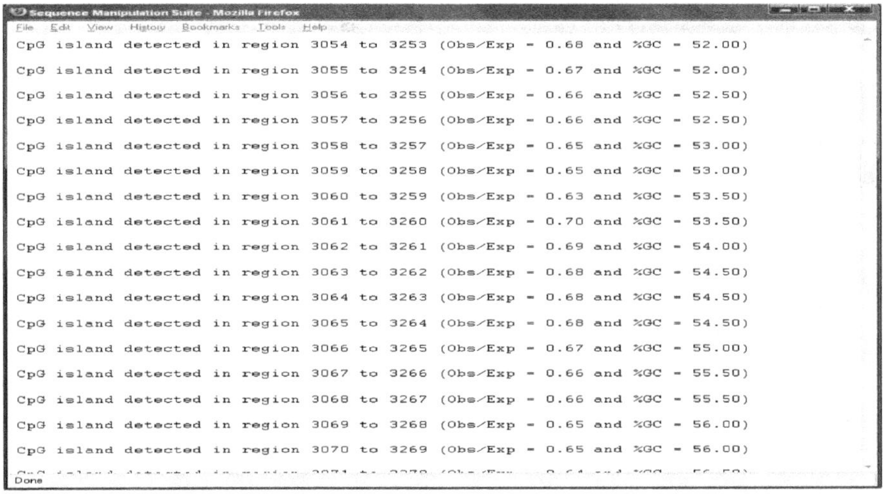

```
Sequence Manipulation Suite - Mozilla Firefox                                    _ □ X
File  Edit  View  History  Bookmarks  Tools  Help

CpG island detected in region 3054 to 3253 (Obs/Exp = 0.68 and %GC = 52.00)

CpG island detected in region 3055 to 3254 (Obs/Exp = 0.67 and %GC = 52.00)

CpG island detected in region 3056 to 3255 (Obs/Exp = 0.66 and %GC = 52.50)

CpG island detected in region 3057 to 3256 (Obs/Exp = 0.66 and %GC = 52.50)

CpG island detected in region 3058 to 3257 (Obs/Exp = 0.65 and %GC = 53.00)

CpG island detected in region 3059 to 3258 (Obs/Exp = 0.65 and %GC = 53.00)

CpG island detected in region 3060 to 3259 (Obs/Exp = 0.63 and %GC = 53.50)

CpG island detected in region 3061 to 3260 (Obs/Exp = 0.70 and %GC = 53.50)

CpG island detected in region 3062 to 3261 (Obs/Exp = 0.69 and %GC = 54.00)

CpG island detected in region 3063 to 3262 (Obs/Exp = 0.68 and %GC = 54.50)

CpG island detected in region 3064 to 3263 (Obs/Exp = 0.68 and %GC = 54.50)

CpG island detected in region 3065 to 3264 (Obs/Exp = 0.68 and %GC = 54.50)

CpG island detected in region 3066 to 3265 (Obs/Exp = 0.67 and %GC = 55.00)

CpG island detected in region 3067 to 3266 (Obs/Exp = 0.66 and %GC = 55.50)

CpG island detected in region 3068 to 3267 (Obs/Exp = 0.66 and %GC = 55.50)

CpG island detected in region 3069 to 3268 (Obs/Exp = 0.65 and %GC = 56.00)

CpG island detected in region 3070 to 3269 (Obs/Exp = 0.65 and %GC = 56.00)

CpG island detected in region 3071 to 3270 (Obs/Exp = 0.64 and %GC = 56.50)
Done
```

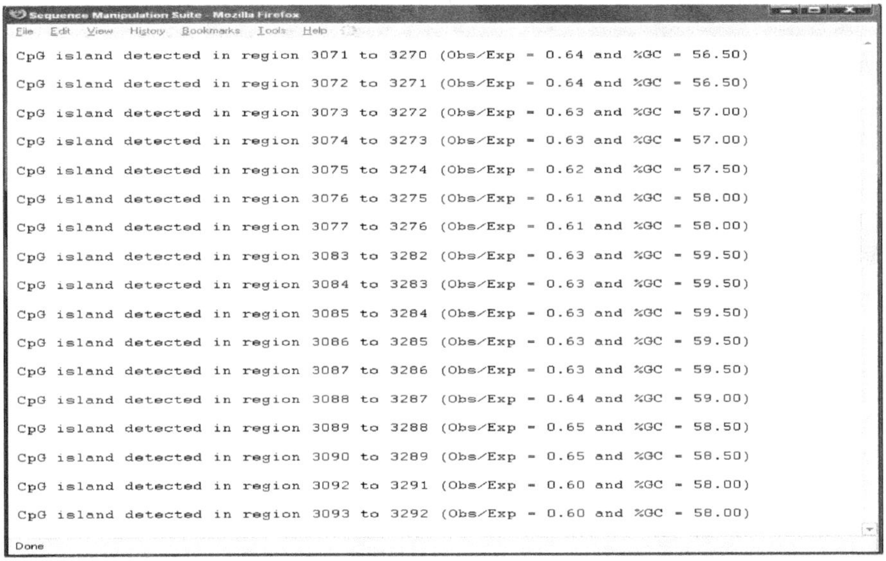

```
Sequence Manipulation Suite - Mozilla Firefox                                    _ □ X
File  Edit  View  History  Bookmarks  Tools  Help

CpG island detected in region 3071 to 3270 (Obs/Exp = 0.64 and %GC = 56.50)

CpG island detected in region 3072 to 3271 (Obs/Exp = 0.64 and %GC = 56.50)

CpG island detected in region 3073 to 3272 (Obs/Exp = 0.63 and %GC = 57.00)

CpG island detected in region 3074 to 3273 (Obs/Exp = 0.63 and %GC = 57.00)

CpG island detected in region 3075 to 3274 (Obs/Exp = 0.62 and %GC = 57.50)

CpG island detected in region 3076 to 3275 (Obs/Exp = 0.61 and %GC = 58.00)

CpG island detected in region 3077 to 3276 (Obs/Exp = 0.61 and %GC = 58.00)

CpG island detected in region 3083 to 3282 (Obs/Exp = 0.63 and %GC = 59.50)

CpG island detected in region 3084 to 3283 (Obs/Exp = 0.63 and %GC = 59.50)

CpG island detected in region 3085 to 3284 (Obs/Exp = 0.63 and %GC = 59.50)

CpG island detected in region 3086 to 3285 (Obs/Exp = 0.63 and %GC = 59.50)

CpG island detected in region 3087 to 3286 (Obs/Exp = 0.63 and %GC = 59.50)

CpG island detected in region 3088 to 3287 (Obs/Exp = 0.64 and %GC = 59.00)

CpG island detected in region 3089 to 3288 (Obs/Exp = 0.65 and %GC = 58.50)

CpG island detected in region 3090 to 3289 (Obs/Exp = 0.65 and %GC = 58.50)

CpG island detected in region 3092 to 3291 (Obs/Exp = 0.60 and %GC = 58.00)

CpG island detected in region 3093 to 3292 (Obs/Exp = 0.60 and %GC = 58.00)
Done
```

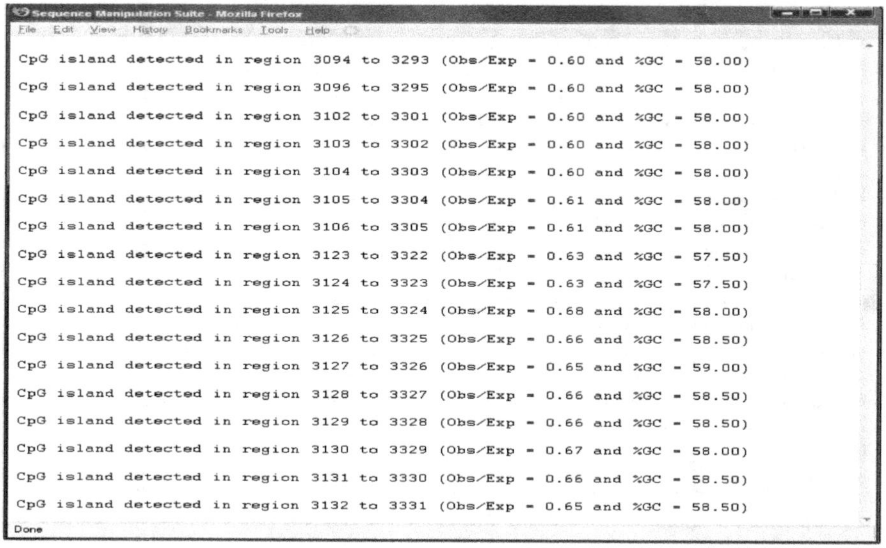

```
Sequence Manipulation Suite - Mozilla Firefox
File  Edit  View  History  Bookmarks  Tools  Help

CpG island detected in region 3094 to 3293 (Obs/Exp = 0.60 and %GC = 58.00)
CpG island detected in region 3096 to 3295 (Obs/Exp = 0.60 and %GC = 58.00)
CpG island detected in region 3102 to 3301 (Obs/Exp = 0.60 and %GC = 58.00)
CpG island detected in region 3103 to 3302 (Obs/Exp = 0.60 and %GC = 58.00)
CpG island detected in region 3104 to 3303 (Obs/Exp = 0.60 and %GC = 58.00)
CpG island detected in region 3105 to 3304 (Obs/Exp = 0.61 and %GC = 58.00)
CpG island detected in region 3106 to 3305 (Obs/Exp = 0.61 and %GC = 58.00)
CpG island detected in region 3123 to 3322 (Obs/Exp = 0.63 and %GC = 57.50)
CpG island detected in region 3124 to 3323 (Obs/Exp = 0.63 and %GC = 57.50)
CpG island detected in region 3125 to 3324 (Obs/Exp = 0.68 and %GC = 58.00)
CpG island detected in region 3126 to 3325 (Obs/Exp = 0.66 and %GC = 58.50)
CpG island detected in region 3127 to 3326 (Obs/Exp = 0.65 and %GC = 59.00)
CpG island detected in region 3128 to 3327 (Obs/Exp = 0.66 and %GC = 58.50)
CpG island detected in region 3129 to 3328 (Obs/Exp = 0.66 and %GC = 58.50)
CpG island detected in region 3130 to 3329 (Obs/Exp = 0.67 and %GC = 58.00)
CpG island detected in region 3131 to 3330 (Obs/Exp = 0.66 and %GC = 58.50)
CpG island detected in region 3132 to 3331 (Obs/Exp = 0.65 and %GC = 58.50)
Done
```

```
Sequence Manipulation Suite - Mozilla Firefox
File  Edit  View  History  Bookmarks  Tools  Help

CpG island detected in region 3133 to 3332 (Obs/Exp = 0.66 and %GC = 58.00)
CpG island detected in region 3134 to 3333 (Obs/Exp = 0.66 and %GC = 58.00)
CpG island detected in region 3135 to 3334 (Obs/Exp = 0.68 and %GC = 57.50)
CpG island detected in region 3136 to 3335 (Obs/Exp = 0.66 and %GC = 58.00)
CpG island detected in region 3137 to 3336 (Obs/Exp = 0.65 and %GC = 58.50)
CpG island detected in region 3138 to 3337 (Obs/Exp = 0.71 and %GC = 58.50)
CpG island detected in region 3139 to 3338 (Obs/Exp = 0.71 and %GC = 58.50)
CpG island detected in region 3140 to 3339 (Obs/Exp = 0.70 and %GC = 59.00)
CpG island detected in region 3141 to 3340 (Obs/Exp = 0.69 and %GC = 59.00)
CpG island detected in region 3142 to 3341 (Obs/Exp = 0.71 and %GC = 58.50)
CpG island detected in region 3143 to 3342 (Obs/Exp = 0.71 and %GC = 58.50)
CpG island detected in region 3144 to 3343 (Obs/Exp = 0.72 and %GC = 58.00)
CpG island detected in region 3145 to 3344 (Obs/Exp = 0.73 and %GC = 57.50)
CpG island detected in region 3146 to 3345 (Obs/Exp = 0.73 and %GC = 57.50)
CpG island detected in region 3147 to 3346 (Obs/Exp = 0.73 and %GC = 57.50)
CpG island detected in region 3148 to 3347 (Obs/Exp = 0.72 and %GC = 58.00)
CpG island detected in region 3149 to 3348 (Obs/Exp = 0.73 and %GC = 57.50)
Done
```

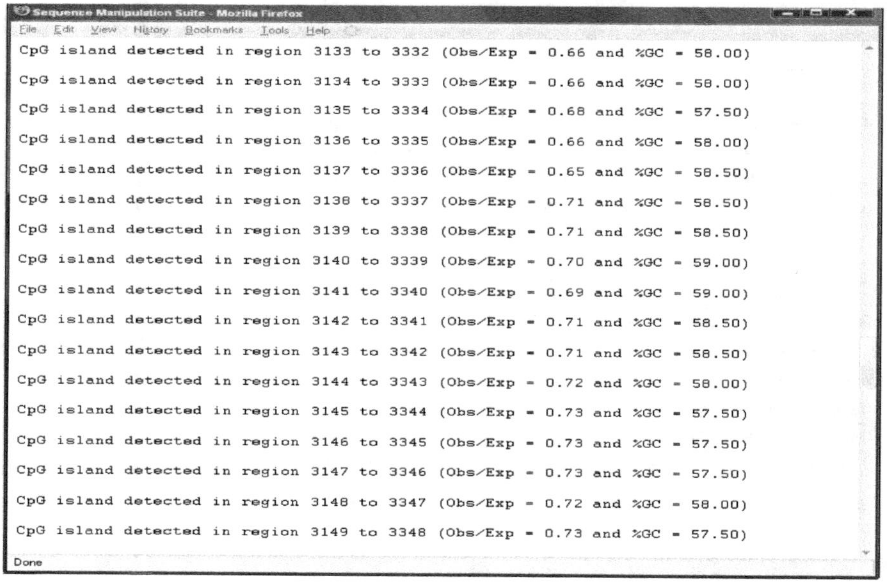

CpG island detected in region 3150 to 3349 (Obs/Exp = 0.72 and %GC = 58.00)

CpG island detected in region 3151 to 3350 (Obs/Exp = 0.73 and %GC = 57.50)

CpG island detected in region 3152 to 3351 (Obs/Exp = 0.72 and %GC = 58.00)

CpG island detected in region 3153 to 3352 (Obs/Exp = 0.71 and %GC = 58.50)

CpG island detected in region 3154 to 3353 (Obs/Exp = 0.76 and %GC = 58.50)

CpG island detected in region 3155 to 3354 (Obs/Exp = 0.78 and %GC = 58.00)

CpG island detected in region 3156 to 3355 (Obs/Exp = 0.76 and %GC = 58.50)

CpG island detected in region 3157 to 3356 (Obs/Exp = 0.78 and %GC = 58.00)

CpG island detected in region 3158 to 3357 (Obs/Exp = 0.78 and %GC = 58.00)

CpG island detected in region 3159 to 3358 (Obs/Exp = 0.79 and %GC = 57.50)

CpG island detected in region 3160 to 3359 (Obs/Exp = 0.78 and %GC = 58.00)

CpG island detected in region 3161 to 3360 (Obs/Exp = 0.76 and %GC = 58.50)

CpG island detected in region 3162 to 3361 (Obs/Exp = 0.82 and %GC = 58.50)

CpG island detected in region 3163 to 3362 (Obs/Exp = 0.82 and %GC = 58.50)

CpG island detected in region 3164 to 3363 (Obs/Exp = 0.81 and %GC = 59.00)

CpG island detected in region 3165 to 3364 (Obs/Exp = 0.82 and %GC = 58.50)

CpG island detected in region 3166 to 3365 (Obs/Exp = 0.83 and %GC = 58.00)

Done

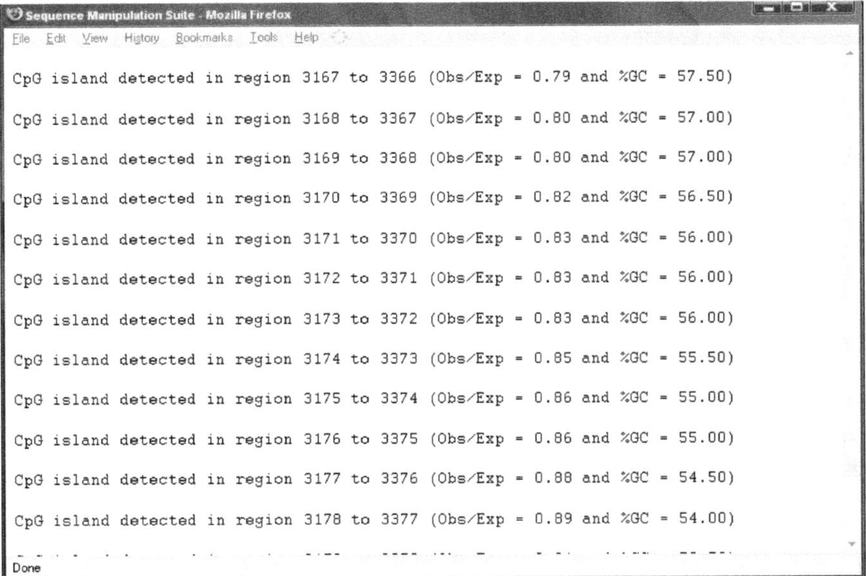

CpG island detected in region 3167 to 3366 (Obs/Exp = 0.79 and %GC = 57.50)

CpG island detected in region 3168 to 3367 (Obs/Exp = 0.80 and %GC = 57.00)

CpG island detected in region 3169 to 3368 (Obs/Exp = 0.80 and %GC = 57.00)

CpG island detected in region 3170 to 3369 (Obs/Exp = 0.82 and %GC = 56.50)

CpG island detected in region 3171 to 3370 (Obs/Exp = 0.83 and %GC = 56.00)

CpG island detected in region 3172 to 3371 (Obs/Exp = 0.83 and %GC = 56.00)

CpG island detected in region 3173 to 3372 (Obs/Exp = 0.83 and %GC = 56.00)

CpG island detected in region 3174 to 3373 (Obs/Exp = 0.85 and %GC = 55.50)

CpG island detected in region 3175 to 3374 (Obs/Exp = 0.86 and %GC = 55.00)

CpG island detected in region 3176 to 3375 (Obs/Exp = 0.86 and %GC = 55.00)

CpG island detected in region 3177 to 3376 (Obs/Exp = 0.88 and %GC = 54.50)

CpG island detected in region 3178 to 3377 (Obs/Exp = 0.89 and %GC = 54.00)

Done

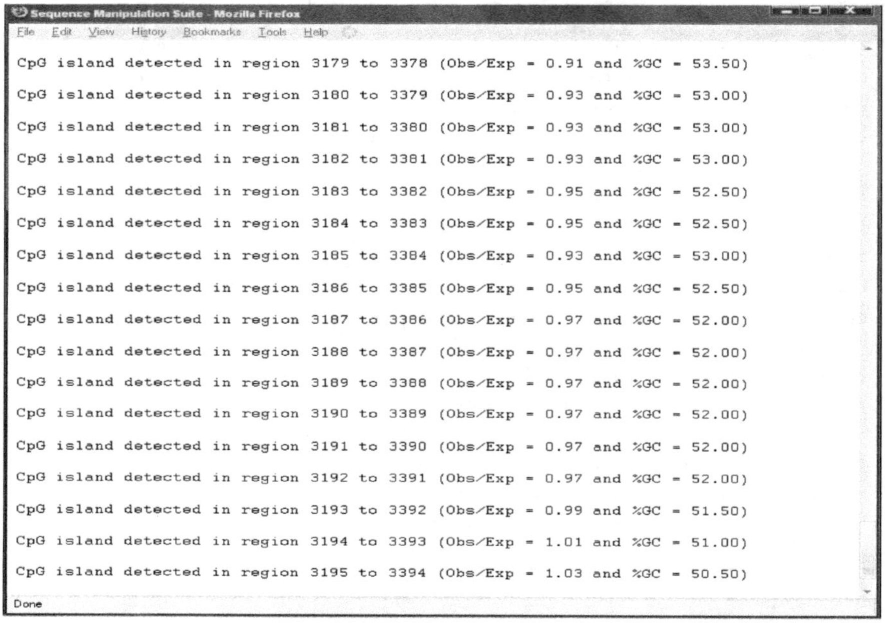

CpG island detected in region 3179 to 3378 (Obs/Exp = 0.91 and %GC = 53.50)

CpG island detected in region 3180 to 3379 (Obs/Exp = 0.93 and %GC = 53.00)

CpG island detected in region 3181 to 3380 (Obs/Exp = 0.93 and %GC = 53.00)

CpG island detected in region 3182 to 3381 (Obs/Exp = 0.93 and %GC = 53.00)

CpG island detected in region 3183 to 3382 (Obs/Exp = 0.95 and %GC = 52.50)

CpG island detected in region 3184 to 3383 (Obs/Exp = 0.95 and %GC = 52.50)

CpG island detected in region 3185 to 3384 (Obs/Exp = 0.93 and %GC = 53.00)

CpG island detected in region 3186 to 3385 (Obs/Exp = 0.95 and %GC = 52.50)

CpG island detected in region 3187 to 3386 (Obs/Exp = 0.97 and %GC = 52.00)

CpG island detected in region 3188 to 3387 (Obs/Exp = 0.97 and %GC = 52.00)

CpG island detected in region 3189 to 3388 (Obs/Exp = 0.97 and %GC = 52.00)

CpG island detected in region 3190 to 3389 (Obs/Exp = 0.97 and %GC = 52.00)

CpG island detected in region 3191 to 3390 (Obs/Exp = 0.97 and %GC = 52.00)

CpG island detected in region 3192 to 3391 (Obs/Exp = 0.97 and %GC = 52.00)

CpG island detected in region 3193 to 3392 (Obs/Exp = 0.99 and %GC = 51.50)

CpG island detected in region 3194 to 3393 (Obs/Exp = 1.01 and %GC = 51.00)

CpG island detected in region 3195 to 3394 (Obs/Exp = 1.03 and %GC = 50.50)

4

PROTEIN STRUCTURE PREDICTION

1. PROTEIN STRUCTURE PREDICTION

Protein structure prediction is the prediction of the three-dimensional structure of a protein from its amino acid sequence—that is, the prediction of a protein's tertiary structure from its primary structure. It is one of the most important goals pursued by bioinformatics and theoretical chemistry.

With no homologue of known structure from which to make a 3D model, a logical next step is to predict secondary structure. Although they differ in method, the aim of secondary structure prediction is to provide the location of alpha helices, and beta strands within a protein or protein family.

There are now many web servers for structure prediction, here is quick summary:

- *PSI-pred* (PSI-BLAST profiles used for prediction; David Jones, Warwick)
- *JPRED* Consensus prediction (includes many of the methods given below; Cuff & Barton, EBI)
- *DSC* King & Sternberg (this server)
- PREDATORFrischman & Argos (EMBL)
- *PHD home page* Rost & Sander, EMBL, Germany
- *ZPRED server* Zvelebil et al., Ludwig, U.K.
- *nnPredict* Cohen et al., UCSF, USA.
- *BMERC PSA Server* Boston University, USA
- *SSP (Nearest-neighbor)* Solovyev and Salamov, Baylor College, USA.

Methods for single sequences

Secondary structure prediction has been around for almost a quarter of a century. The early methods suffered from a lack of data. Predictions were performed on single sequences rather than families of homologous sequences, and there were relatively few known 3D structures from which to derive parameters. Probably the most famous early methods are those of Chou & Fasman, Garnier, Osguthorbe & Robson (GOR) and Lim. Although the authors originally claimed quite high accuracies (70-80 %), under careful examination, the methods were shown to be only between 56 and 60% accurate (see Kabsch & Sander, 1984 given below). An early problem in secondary structure prediction had been the inclusion of structures used to derive parameters in the set of structures, used to assess the accuracy of the method.

Comparative protein modelling uses previously solved structures as starting points, or templates. This is effective because, it appears that although the number of actual proteins is vast, there is a limited set of tertiary structural motifs to which most proteins belong. It has been suggested that there are only around 2000 distinct protein folds in nature, though there are many millions of different proteins.

These methods may also be split into two groups [1]:

- *Homology modeling* is based on the reasonable assumption that two *homologous* proteins will share very similar structures. Because a protein's fold is more evolutionarily conserved than its amino acid sequence, a target sequence (the structure of protein is yet solved)can be modeled with reasonable accuracy on a very distantly related template (protein structure is solved experimentally-x-ray/NMR), provided that the relationship between target and template can be discerned through *sequence alignment.* It has been suggested that the primary bottleneck in comparative modelling arises from difficulties in alignment rather than from errors in structure prediction, gives a known-good alignment.

- *Protein threading* scans the amino acid sequence of an unknown structure against a database of solved structures. In each case, a scoring function is used to assess the compatibility of the sequence to the structure, thus yielding possible three-dimensional models. This type of method is also known as **3D-1D fold recognition** due to its compatibility analysis between three-dimensional structures and linear protein sequences. This method has also given rise to methods performing an **inverse folding search** by evaluating the compatibility of a given structure with a large database of sequences, thus predicting which sequences have the potential to produce a given fold.

Exercise: 12

SECONDARY STRUCTURE PREDICTION OF A PROTEIN

GOR IV Algorithm

Aim: To predict secondary structure of human cox 2 using GOR-IV algorithm.

Procedure

* Retrieve protein sequence from NCBI database in FASTA format.
* Login to
  http://npsa-pbil.ibcp.fr/cgi-bin/npsa_automat.pl?page=npsa_gor4.html to perform secondary structure prediction.
* Paste the protein sequence in the input box.
* Submit the procedure by clicking on SUBMIT button.
* Result will be obtained after the completion of the task.

Results and Discussion

Results were obtained representing secondary structure elements with their single letter codes such as Helix-h, Beta sheets–e,Coils-c.

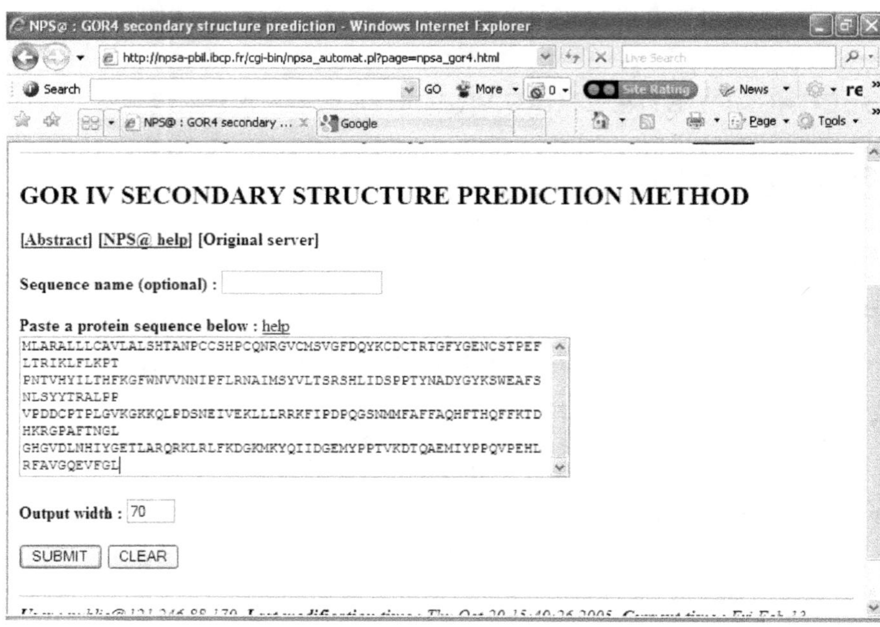

NPS@ : GOR4 secondary structure prediction - Windows Internet Explorer
http://npsa-pbil.ibcp.fr/cgi-bin/npsa_automat.pl?page=npsa_gor4.html
Live Search
Search
GO   More   0
Site Rating   News   re
NPS@ : GOR4 secondary ...   Google
Page   Tools
GOR IV SECONDARY STRUCTURE PREDICTION METHOD
[Abstract] [NPS@ help] [Original server]
Sequence name (optional) :
Paste a protein sequence below : help
MLARALLLCAVLALSHTANPCCSHPCQNRGVCMSVGFDQYKCDCTRTGFYGENCSTPEF
LTRIKLFLKPT
PNTVHYILTHFKGFWNVVNNIPFLRNAIMSYVLTSRSHLIDSPPTYNADYGYKSWEAFS
NLSYYTRALPP
VPDDCPTPLGVKGKKQLPDSNEIVEKLLLRRKFIPDPQGSNMMFAFFAQHFTHQFFKTD
HKRGPAFTNGL
GHGVDLNHIYGETLARQRKLRLFKDGKMKYQIIDGEMYPPTVKDTQAEMIYPPQVPEHL
RFAVGQEVFGL
Output width : 70
SUBMIT   CLEAR

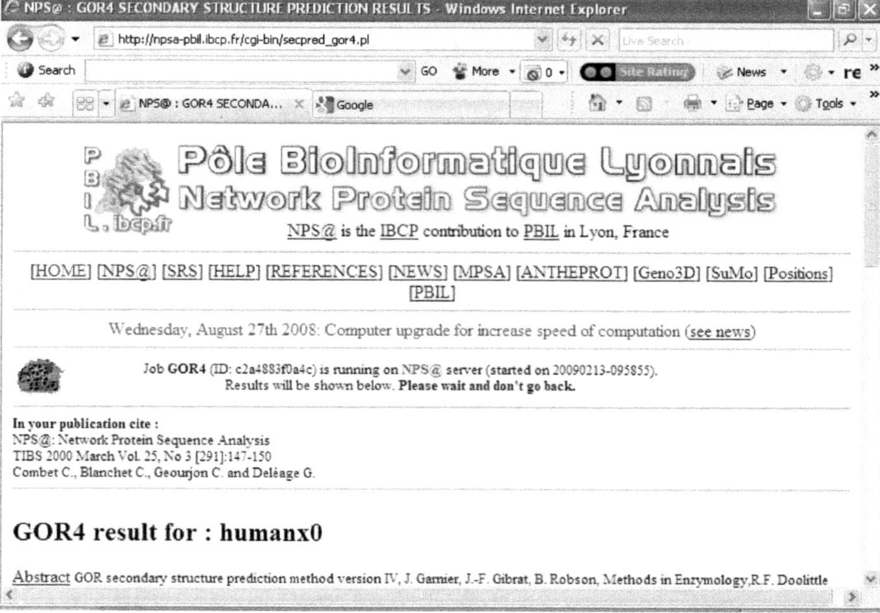

NPS@ : GOR4 SECONDARY STRUCTURE PREDICTION RESULTS - Windows Internet Explorer
http://npsa-pbil.ibcp.fr/cgi-bin/secpred_gor4.pl
Live Search
Search
GO   More   0
Site Rating   News   re
NPS@ : GOR4 SECONDA...   Google
Page   Tools
P
B
I
L , ibcp.fr
Pôle BioInformatique Lyonnais
Network Protein Sequence Analysis
NPS@ is the IBCP contribution to PBIL in Lyon, France
[HOME] [NPS@] [SRS] [HELP] [REFERENCES] [NEWS] [MPSA] [ANTHEPROT] [Geno3D] [SuMo] [Positions] [PBIL]
Wednesday, August 27th 2008: Computer upgrade for increase speed of computation (see news)
Job GOR4 (ID: c2a4883f0a4c) is running on NPS@ server (started on 20090213-095855).
Results will be shown below. Please wait and don't go back.
In your publication cite :
NPS@: Network Protein Sequence Analysis
TIBS 2000 March Vol. 25, No 3 [291]:147-150
Combet C., Blanchet C., Geourjon C. and Deléage G.
GOR4 result for : humanx0
Abstract GOR secondary structure prediction method version IV, J. Garnier, J.-F. Gibrat, B. Robson, Methods in Enzymology,R.F. Doolittle

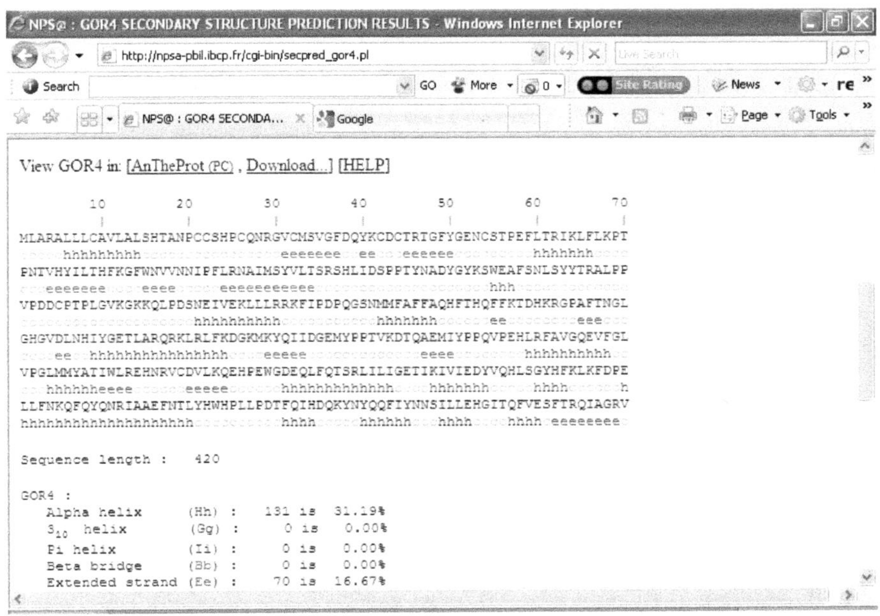

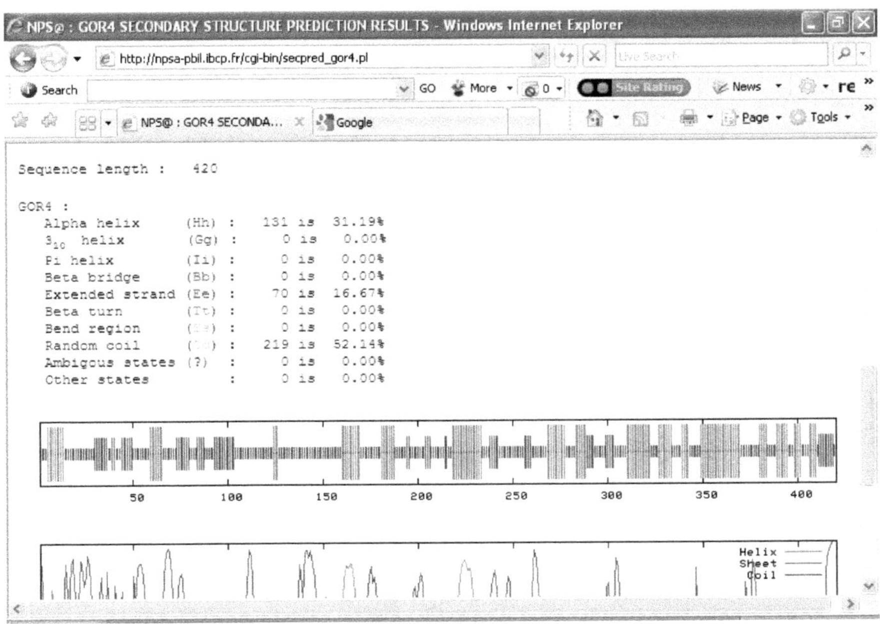

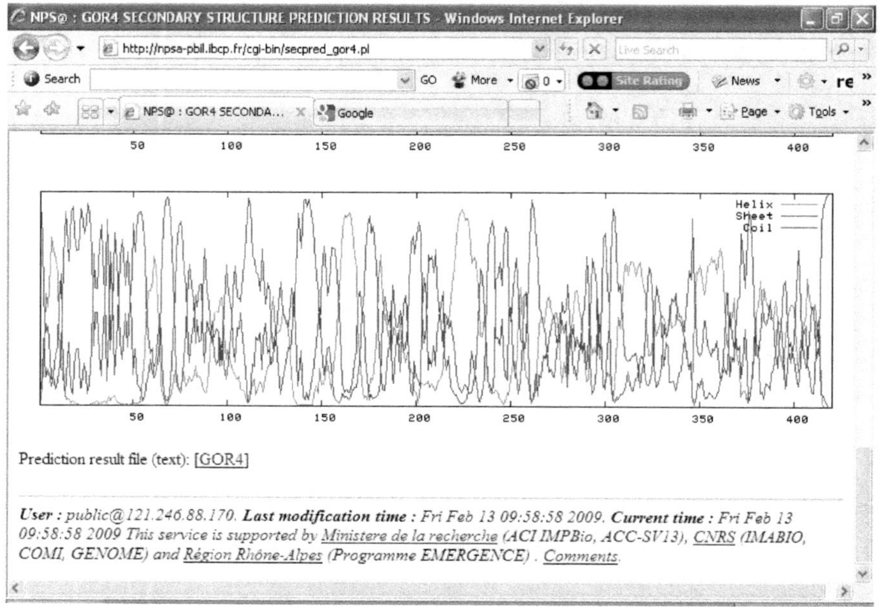

Exercise: 13

JMPred

Aim: To predict secondary structure of human cox 2 usingJPred software.

Procedure

* Retrieve protein sequence from NCBI database in FASTA format.
* Login to http://www.compbio.dundee.ac.uk/~www-jpred/
* to perform secondary structure prediction.
* Paste the protein sequence in the input box.
* Submit the procedure by clicking on MAKE PREDICTION button.
* Result will be obtained after the completion of the task.

Result and Discussion

Results were obtained representing secondary structure elements with their single letter codes such as Helix-h, Beta sheets–e.

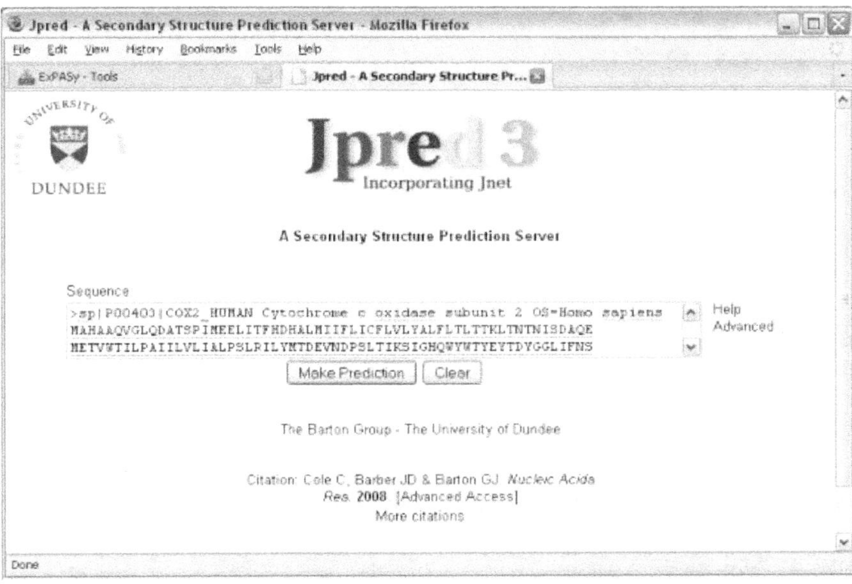

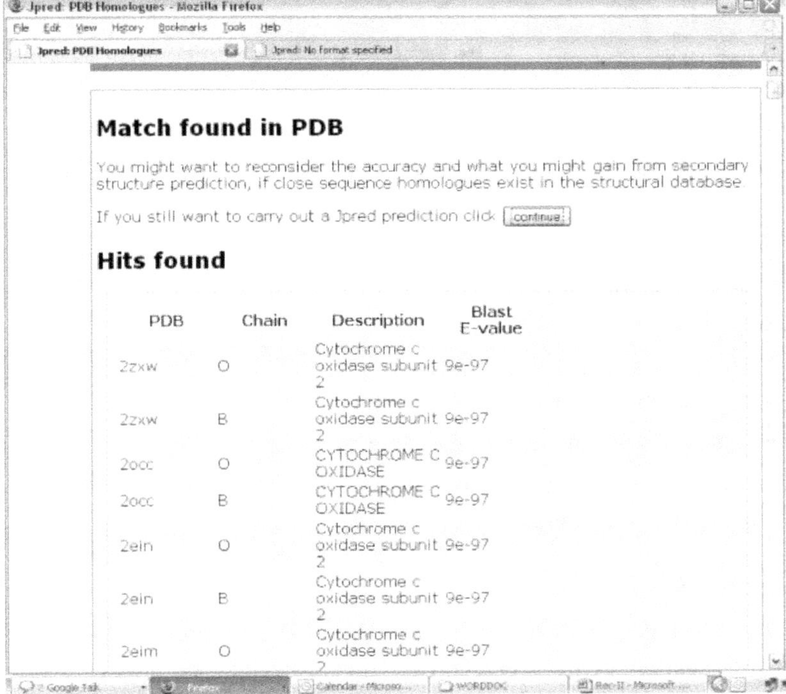

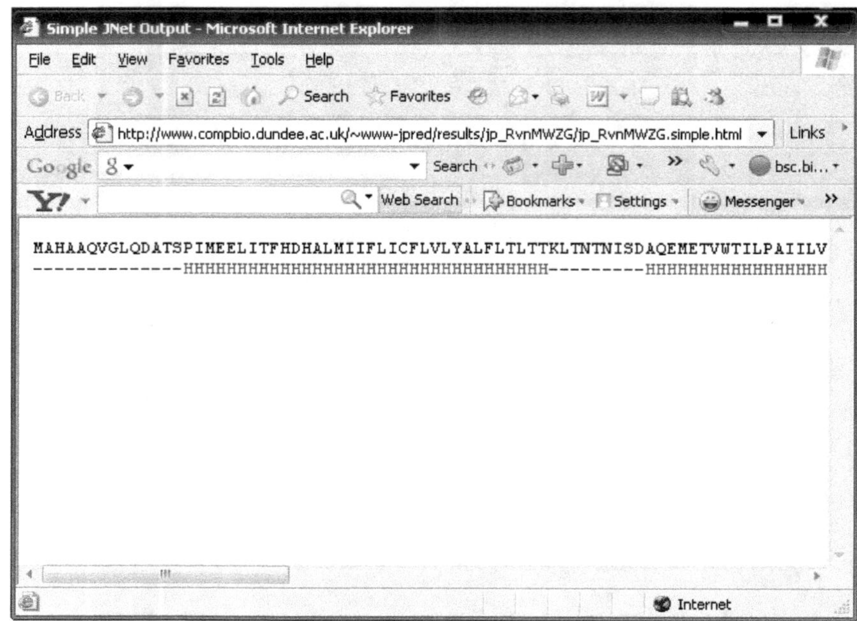

Exercise: 14

SOPMA

Aim: To predict secondary structure of human Cox 2 using SOPMA.

Procedure

- Retrieve protein sequence from NCBI database in FASTA format
- .Login to
  http://npsa-pbil.ibcp.fr/cgi-in/npsa_automat.pl?page=npsa_sopma.html to perform secondary structure prediction.
- Paste the protein sequence in the input box.
- Submit the procedure by clicking on SUBMIT button. Result will be obtained after the completion of the task.

Result and Discussion

Results were obtained representing secondary structure elements with their single letter codes such as Helix-h, Beta sheets–e, Coils-c.

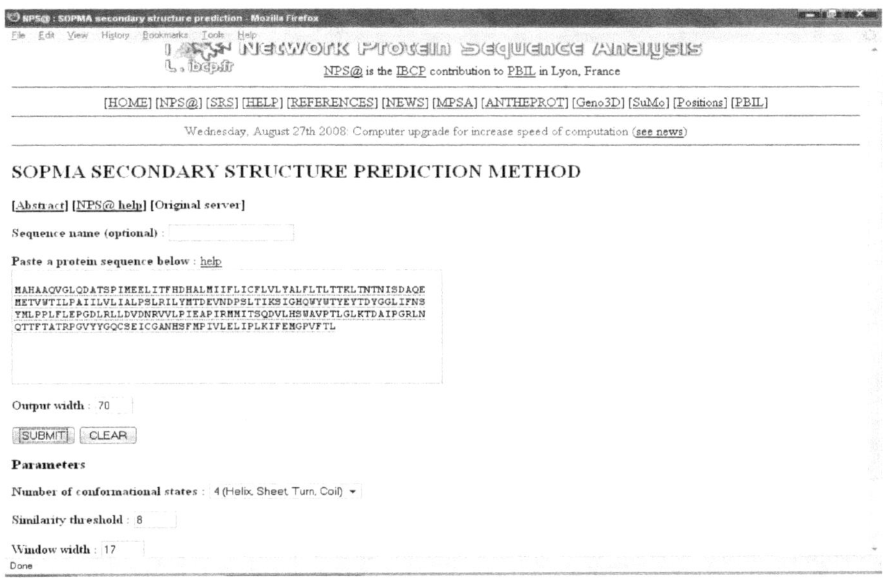

NPS@ : SOPMA secondary structure prediction - Mozilla Firefox
File   Edit   View   History   Bookmarks   Tools   Help
NETWORK PROTEIN SEQUENCE ANALYSIS
NPS@ is the IBCP contribution to PBIL in Lyon, France
[HOME] [NPS@] [SRS] [HELP] [REFERENCES] [NEWS] [MPSA] [ANTHEPROT] [Geno3D] [SuMo] [Positions] [PBIL]
Wednesday, August 27th 2008: Computer upgrade for increase speed of computation (see news)
SOPMA SECONDARY STRUCTURE PREDICTION METHOD
[Abstract] [NPS@ help] [Original server]
Sequence name (optional) :
Paste a protein sequence below : help
MAHAAQVGLQDATSPIMEELITFHDHALMIIFLICFLVLYALFLTLTTKLTNTNISDAQE
METVWTILPAIILVLIALPSLRILYMTDEVNDPSLTIKSIGHQWYWTYEYTDYGGLIFNS
YMLPPLFLEPGDLRLLDVDNRVVLPIEAPIRMMITSQDVLHSWAVPTLGLKTDAIPGRLN
QTTFTATRPGVYYGQCSEICGANHSFMPIVLELIPLKIFEMGPVFTL
Output width : 70
SUBMIT   CLEAR
Parameters
Number of conformational states : 4 (Helix, Sheet, Turn, Coil)
Similarity threshold : 8
Window width : 17
Done

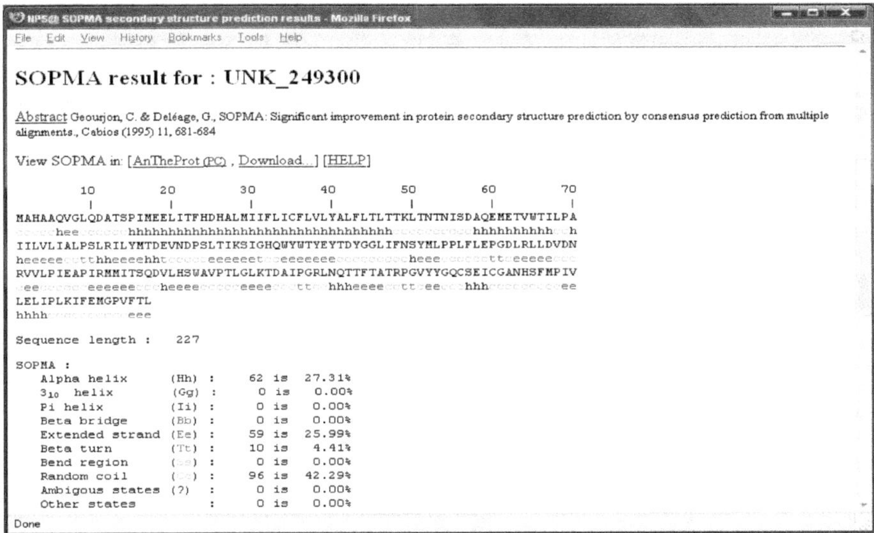

NPS@ SOPMA secondary structure prediction results - Mozilla Firefox
File   Edit   View   History   Bookmarks   Tools   Help
SOPMA result for : UNK_249300
Abstract Geourjon, C. & Deléage, G., SOPMA: Significant improvement in protein secondary structure prediction by consensus prediction from multiple alignments., Cabios (1995) 11, 681-684
View SOPMA in: [AnTheProt (PC) , Download...] [HELP]
         10   20   30   40   50   60   70
          | | | | | | |
MAHAAQVGLQDATSPIMEELITFHDHALMIIFLICFLVLYALFLTLTTKLTNTNISDAQEMETVWTILPA
       hee   hhhhhhhhhhhhhhhhhhhhhhhhhhhhhhhhhhhhh   hhhhhhhhhh   h
IILVLIALPSLRILYMTDEVNDPSLTIKSIGHQWYWTYEYTDYGGLIFNSYMLPPLFLEPGDLRLLDVDN
heeeee   tthheeeehht   eeeeeet   eeeeeee   heee   tt eeeee
RVVLPIEAPIRMMITSQDVLHSWAVPTLGLKTDAIPGRLNQTTFTATRPGVYYGQCSEICGANHSFMPIV
  ee   eeeeee   heeee   eeee   tt hhheeee   tt ee   hhh   ee
LELIPLKIFEMGPVFTL
hhhh   eee

Sequence length :   227

SOPMA :
    Alpha helix   (Hh) :   62 is   27.31%
    3_10 helix   (Gg) :   0 is   0.00%
    Pi helix   (Ii) :   0 is   0.00%
    Beta bridge   (Bb) :   0 is   0.00%
    Extended strand   (Ee) :   59 is   25.99%
    Beta turn   (Tt) :   10 is   4.41%
    Bend region   ( ) :   0 is   0.00%
    Random coil   ( ) :   96 is   42.29%
    Ambigous states   (?) :   0 is   0.00%
    Other states   :   0 is   0.00%
Done

TMPred:

TMpred - Prediction of Transmembrane Regions and Orientation

The TMpred program makes a prediction of membrane-spanning regions and their orientation. The algorithm is based on the statistical analysis of TMbase, a database of naturally occuring transmembrane proteins. The prediction is made using a combination of several weight-matrices for scoring.

K. Hofmann & W. Stoffel (1993)
TMbase - A database of membrane spanning proteins segments
Biol. Chem. Hoppe-Seyler 374,166

For further information see the TMbase and TMpredict documentation.

Usage: Paste your sequence in one of the supported formats into the sequence field below
and press the "Run TMpred" button.
Make sure that the format button (next to the sequence field) shows the correct format
Choose the minimal and maximal length of the hydrophic part of the transmembrane helix

Output format   html   minimum 17   maximum 33
Query title (optional)   leptin
Input sequence format   Plain Text
Query sequence: or ID or AC or GI (see above for valid formats)
TACTTTTCAGGGCATCTTAGCTTCTATTATAGCCACATCCCTTTGAAACAAGATAACTGA
ATAAGAAAATACATAAGACCATAACAGCCAACAGGTGGCAGGACCAGGACTATAGCCCAG
ACCCAGAGCATTACGTGAGCCAGGTAATGAGGGACTGGAACCAGGGAGACCGAGCGCTTT
GGAGTTTCGAGGTAGAGTTTGAAGGAGGTGAGGGATGTGAATTGCCTGCAGAGAGAAGCC
GAAGGTTTGGTGTGTGGAGATGCAGAGGTAAAAGTGTGAGCAGTGAGTTACAGCGAGAGG

Run TMpred   Clear Input

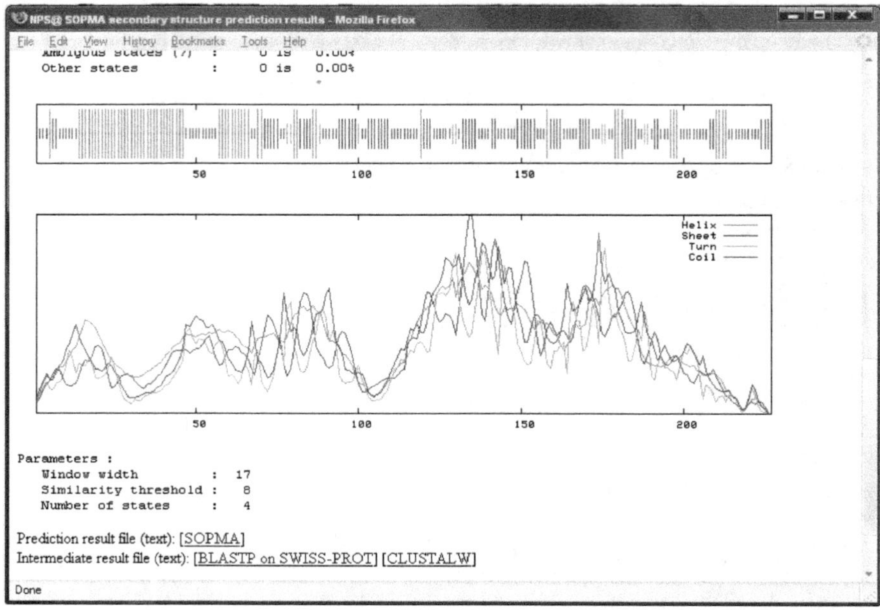

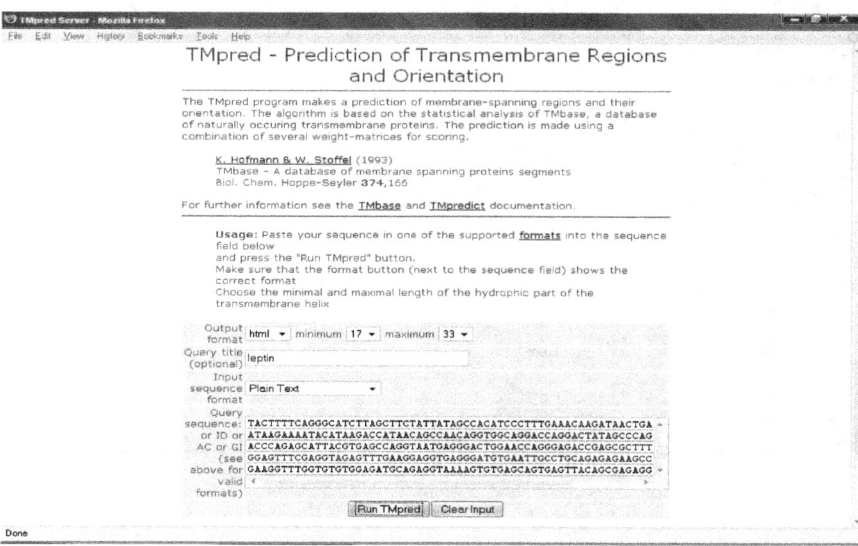

Output

TMpred output for leptin - Mozilla Firefox
File   Edit   View   History   Bookmarks   Tools   Help
min=17 | max=33 | html | leptin | plain_text |
GTAGGAATCGCAGCGCCAGCGGTTGCAAGGCCCAAGAAGCCCATCCTGGGAAGGAAAATGCATTGGGGAA
%0D%0ACCCTGTGCGGATTCTTGTGGCTTTGGCCCTATCTTTTCTATGTCCAAGCTGTGCCCATCCAAAAAGTCCA
%0D%0AAGATGACACCAAAACCCTCATCAAGACAATTGTCACCAGGATCAATGACATTTCACACACGCAGTCAGTC
%0D%0ATCCTCCAAACAGAAAGTCACCGGTTTGGACTTCATTCCTGGGCTCCACCCCATCCTGACCTTATCCAAGA
%0D%0ATGGACCAGACACTGGCAGTCTACCAACAGATCCTCACCAGTATGCCTTCCAGAAACGTGATCCAAATATC
%0D%0ACAACGACCTGGAGAACCTCCGGGATCTTCTTCACGTGCTGGCCTTCTCTAAGAGCTGCCACTTGCCCTGG
%0D%0AGCCAGTGGCCTGGAGACCTTGGACAGCCTGGGGGGTGTCCTGGAAGCTTCAGGCTACTCCACAGAGGTGG
%0D%0ATGGCCCTGAGCAGGCTGCAGGGGTCTCTGCAGGACATGCTGTGGCAGCTGGACCTCAGCCCTGGGTGCTG
%0D%0AAGGCCTTGAAGGTCACTCTTCCTGCAAGGACTACGTTAAGGGAAGGAACTCTGGCTTCCAGGTATCTCCA
%0D%0AGGATTGAAGAGCATTGCATGGACACCCCTTATCCAGGACTCTGTCAATTTCCCTGACTCCTCTAAGCCAC
%0D%0ATCTTCCAAAGGCATAAGACCCTAAGCCTCCTTTTGCTTGAAACCAAAGATATATACACAGGATCCTATTC
%0D%0ATCACCAGGAAGGGGGTCCACCCAGCAAAGAGTGGGCTGCATCTGGGATTCCCACCAAGGTCTTCAGCCAT
%0D%0ACAACAAGAGTTGTCTTGTCCCCTCTTGACCCATCTCCCCCTCACTGAATGCCTCAATGTGACCAGGGGTG
%0D%0AATTTCAGAGAGGGCAGAGGGGTAGGCAGAGCCTTTGGATGACCAGAACAAGGTTCCCTCTGAGAATTCCA
%0D%0AAGGAGTTCCATGAAGACCACATCCACACACGCAGGAACTCCCAGCAACACAAGCTGGAAGCACATGTTTA
%0D%0ATTTATTCTGCATTTTATTCTGGATGGATTTGAAGCAAAGCACCAGCTTCTCCAGGCTCTTTGGGGTCAGC
%0D%0ACAGGGCCAGGGGTCTCCCTGGAGTGCAGTTTCCAATCCCATAGATGGGTCTGGCTGAGCTGAACCCATTT
%0D%0ATGAGTGACTCGAGGGTTGGGTTCATCTGAGCAAGAGCTGGCAAAGGTGGCTCTCCAGTTAGTTCTCTCGT
%0D%0AAAACTGGTTTCATTTCTACTGTGACTGATGTTACATCACAGTGTTTGCAATGGTGTTGCCCTGAGTGGATC
%0D%0ATCCAAGGACCAGGTTATTTTAAAAAGATTTGTTTTGTCAAGTGTCATATGTAGGTGTCTGCACCCAGGGG
%0D%0ATGGGGAATGTTTGGGCAGAAGGGAGAAGGATCTAGAATGTGTTTTCTGAATAACATTTGTGTGGTGGGTT
%0D%0ACTTTGGAAGGAGTGAGATCATTTTCTTATCTTCTGCAATTGCTTAGGATGTTTTTCATGAAAATAGCTCT
%0D%0ATTCAGGGGGGTTGTGAGGCCTGGCCAGGCACCCCCTGGAGAGAAGTTTCTGGCCCTGGCTGACCCCAAAG
%0D%0AAGCCTGGAGAAGCTGATGCTTTGCTTCAAATCCATCCAGAATAAAACGCAAAGGGCTGAAAGCCATTTGT
%0D%0ATGGGGCAGTGGTAAGCTCTGGCTTTCTCCGACTGCTAGGGAGTGGTCTTTCCTATCATGGAGTGACGGTC
%0D%0ACCACACTGGTGACTGCGATCTTCAGAGCAGGGGTCCTTGGTGTGACCCTCTGAATGGTCCAGGGTTGATC
%0D%0AACACTCTGGGTTTATTACATGGCAGTGTTCCTATTTGGGGCTTGCATGCCAAATTGTAGTTCTTGTCTGA
%0D%0ATTGGCTCACCCAAGCAAGGCCAAAATTACCAAAAATCTTGGGGGGTTTTTACTCCAGTGGTGAAGAAAAC
%0D%0ATCCTTTAGCAGGTGGTCCTGAGACCTGACAAGCACTGCTAGGCGAGTGCCAGGACTCCCCAGGCCAGGCC
%0D%0AACCAGGATGGCCCTTCCCACTGGAGGTCACATTCAGGAAGATGAAAGAGGAGGTTTGGGGTCTGCCACCA
%0D%0ATCCTGCTGCTGTGTTTTTGCTATCACACAGTGGGTGGTGGATCTGTCCAAGGAAACTTGAATCAAAGCAG
%0D%0ATTAACTTTAAGACTGAGCACCTGCTTCATGCTCAGCCCTGACTGGTGCTATAGGCTGGAGAAGCTCACCC
Done

TMpred output for leptin - Mozilla Firefox
File   Edit   View   History   Bookmarks   Tools   Help
%0D%0ATGAGTGACTCGAGGGTTGGGTTCATCTGAGCAAGAGCTGGCAAAGGTGGCTCTCCAGTTAGTTCTCTCGT
%0D%0AAAACTGGTTTCATTTCTACTGTGACTGATGTTACATCACAGTGTTTGCAATGGTGTTGCCCTGAGTGGATC
%0D%0ATCCAAGGACCAGGTTATTTTAAAAAGATTTGTTTTGTCAAGTGTCATATGTAGGTGTCTGCACCCAGGGG
%0D%0ATGGGGAATGTTTGGGCAGAAGGGAGAAGGATCTAGAATGTGTTTTCTGAATAACATTTGTGTGGTGGGTT
%0D%0ACTTTGGAAGGAGTGAGATCATTTTCTTATCTTCTGCAATTGCTTAGGATGTTTTTCATGAAAATAGCTCT
%0D%0ATTCAGGGGGGTTGTGAGGCCTGGCCAGGCACCCCCTGGAGAGAAGTTTCTGGCCCTGGCTGACCCCAAAG
%0D%0AAGCCTGGAGAAGCTGATGCTTTGCTTCAAATCCATCCAGAATAAAACGCAAAGGGCTGAAAGCCATTTGT
%0D%0ATGGGGCAGTGGTAAGCTCTGGCTTTCTCCGACTGCTAGGGAGTGGTCTTTCCTATCATGGAGTGACGGTC
%0D%0ACCACACTGGTGACTGCGATCTTCAGAGCAGGGGTCCTTGGTGTGACCCTCTGAATGGTCCAGGGTTGATC
%0D%0AACACTCTGGGTTTATTACATGGCAGTGTTCCTATTTGGGGCTTGCATGCCAAATTGTAGTTCTTGTCTGA
%0D%0ATTGGCTCACCCAAGCAAGGCCAAAATTACCAAAAATCTTGGGGGGTTTTTACTCCAGTGGTGAAGAAAAC
%0D%0ATCCTTTAGCAGGTGGTCCTGAGACCTGACAAGCACTGCTAGGCGAGTGCCAGGACTCCCCAGGCCAGGCC
%0D%0AACCAGGATGGCCCTTCCCACTGGAGGTCACATTCAGGAAGATGAAAGAGGAGGTTTGGGGTCTGCCACCA
%0D%0ATCCTGCTGCTGTGTTTTTGCTATCACACAGTGGGTGGTGGATCTGTCCAAGGAAACTTGAATCAAAGCAG
%0D%0ATTAACTTTAAGACTGAGCACCTGCTTCATGCTCAGCCCTGACTGGTGCTATAGGCTGGAGAAGCTCACCC
%0D%0AAAATAAACATTAAGATTGAGGCCTGCCCTCAGGGATCTTGCATTCCCAGTGGTCAAACCGCACTCACCCAT
%0D%0AGTGCCAAGGTGGGGTATTTACCACAGCAGCTGAACAGCCAAATGCATGGTGCAGTTGACAGCAGGTGGGA
%0D%0AAAATGGTATGAGCTGAGGGGGGCCGTGCCCAGGGGCCCACAGGGAACCCTGCTTGCACTTTGTAACATGTT
%0D%0ATACTTTTCAGGGCATCTTAGCTTCTATTATAGCCACATCCCTTTGAAACAAGATAACTGAGAATTTAAAA
%0D%0AATAAGAAAATACATAAGACCATAACAGCCAACAGGTGGCAGGACCAGGACTATAGCCCAGGTCCTCTGAT
%0D%0AACCCAGAGCATTACGTGAGCCAGGTAATGAGGGACTGGAACCAGGGAGACCGAGCGCTTTCTGGAAAAGA
%0D%0AGGAGTTTCGAGGTAGAGTTTGAAGGAGGTGAGGGATGTGAATTGCCTGCAGAGAGAAGCCTGTTTTGTTG
%0D%0AGAAGGTTTGGTGTGTGGAGATGCAGAGGTAAAAGTGTGAGCAGTGAGTTACAGCGAGAGGCAGAGAAAGA
%0D%0AAGAGACAGGAGGGCAAGGGCCATGCTGAAGGGACCTTGAAGGGTAAAGAAGTTTGATATTAAAGGAGTTA
%0D%0AAGAGTAGCAAGTTCTAGAGAAGAGGCTGGTGCTGTGGCCAGGGTGAGAGCTGCTCTGGAAAATGTGACCC
%0D%0AAGATCCTCACAACCACCTAATCAGGCTGAGGTGTCTTAAGCCTTTTGCTCACAAAACCTGGCACAATGGC
%0D%0ATAATTCCCAGAGTGTGAAACTTCCTAAGTATAAATGGTTGTCTGTTTTTGTAACTTAAAAAAAAAAAAAA
%0D%0AAAGTTTGGCCGGGTGCGGTGGCTCACGCCTGTAATCCCAGCACTTTGGGAGGCCAAGGTGGGGGGATCAC
%0D%0AAAAGGTCACTAGATGGCGAGCATCCTGGCCAACATGGTGAAACCCCGTCTCTACTAAAAACACAAAAGTTA
%0D%0AGCTGAGCGTGGTGGCGGGCGCCTGTAGTCCCAGCCACTCGGGAGGCTGAGACAGGAGAATCGCTTAAACC
%0D%0ATGGGAGGCGGAGAGTACAGTGAGCCAAGATCGCGCCACTGCACTCCGGCCTGATGACAGAGCGAGATTCC
%0D%0AGTCTTAAAAAAAAAAAAAAAAAAAAGTTTGTTTTTAAAAAAATCTAAATAAAATAACTTTGCCCCCTGCAAA
%0D%0AAAAAAAAAAAAAAAAA%0D%0A%0D%0A
Done

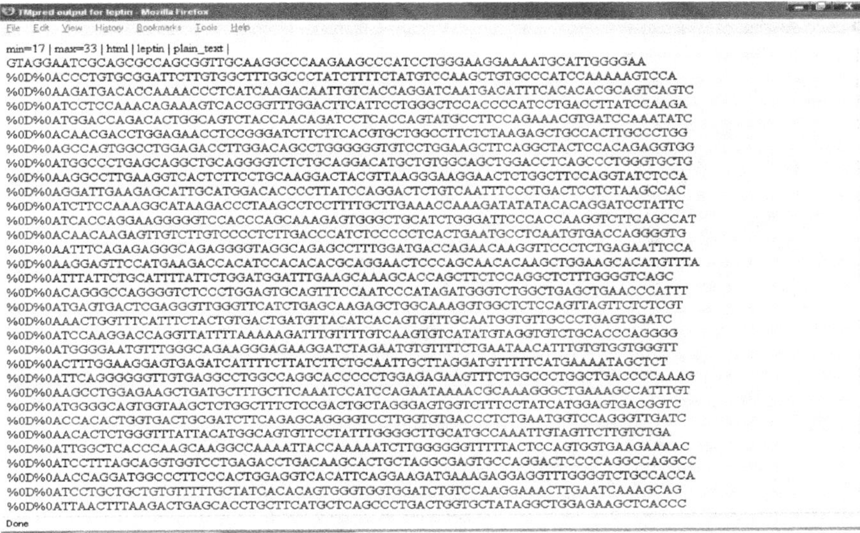

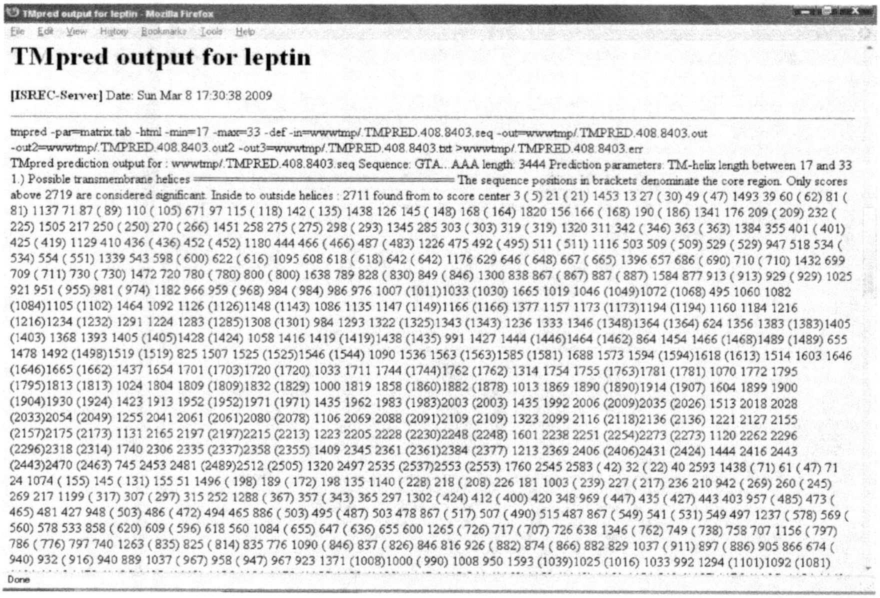

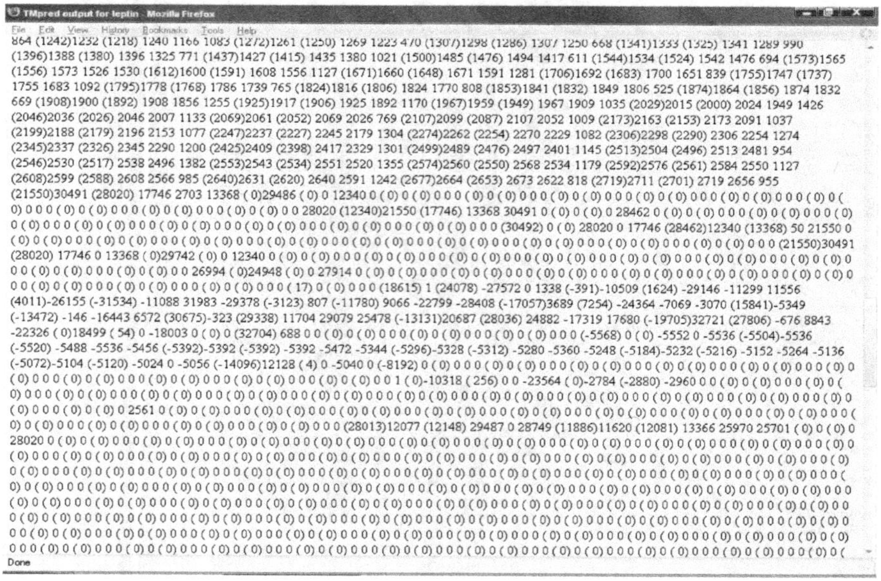

TMpred output for leptin

[ISREC-Server] Date: Sun Mar 8 17:30:38 2009

tmpred -par=matrix.tab -html -min=17 -max=33 -def -in=wwwtmp/.TMPRED.408.8403.seq -out=wwwtmp/.TMPRED.408.8403.out -out2=wwwtmp/.TMPRED.408.8403.out2 -out3=wwwtmp/.TMPRED.408.8403.txt >wwwtmp/.TMPRED.408.8403.err

TMpred prediction output for : wwwtmp/.TMPRED.408.8403.seq Sequence: GTA...AAA length: 3444 Prediction parameters: TM-helix length between 17 and 33

1.) Possible transmembrane helices ======================= The sequence positions in brackets denominate the core region. Only scores above 2719 are considered significant. Inside to outside helices : 2711 found from to score center 3 (5) 21 (21) 1453 13 27 (30) 49 (47) 1493 39 60 (62) 81 (81) 1137 71 87 (89) 110 (105) 671 97 115 (118) 142 (135) 1438 126 145 (148) 168 (164) 1820 156 166 (168) 190 (186) 1341 176 209 (209) 232 (225) 1505 217 250 (250) 270 (266) 1451 258 275 (275) 298 (293) 1345 285 303 (303) 319 (319) 1320 311 342 (346) 363 (363) 1384 355 401 (401) 425 (419) 1129 410 436 (436) 452 (452) 1180 444 466 (466) 487 (483) 1226 475 492 (495) 511 (511) 1116 503 509 (509) 529 (529) 947 518 534 (534) 554 (551) 1339 543 598 (600) 622 (616) 1095 608 618 (618) 642 (642) 1176 629 646 (648) 667 (665) 1396 657 686 (690) 710 (710) 1432 699 709 (711) 730 (730) 1472 720 780 (780) 800 (800) 1638 789 828 (830) 849 (846) 1300 838 867 (867) 887 (887) 1584 877 913 (913) 929 (929) 1025 921 951 (955) 981 (974) 1182 966 959 (968) 984 (984) 986 976 1007 (1011)1033 (1030) 1665 1019 1046 (1049)1072 (1068) 495 1060 1082 (1084)1105 (1102) 1464 1092 1126 (1126)1148 (1143) 1086 1135 1147 (1149)1166 (1166) 1377 1157 1173 (1173)1194 (1194) 1160 1184 1216 (1216)1234 (1232) 1291 1224 1283 (1285)1308 (1301) 984 1293 1322 (1325)1343 (1343) 1236 1333 1346 (1348)1364 (1364) 624 1356 1383 (1383)1405 (1403) 1368 1393 1405 (1405)1428 (1424) 1058 1416 1419 (1419)1438 (1435) 991 1427 1444 (1446)1464 (1462) 864 1454 1466 (1468)1489 (1489) 655 1478 1492 (1498)1519 (1519) 825 1507 1525 (1525)1546 (1544) 1090 1536 1563 (1563)1585 (1581) 1688 1573 1594 (1594)1618 (1613) 1514 1603 1646 (1646)1665 (1662) 1437 1654 1701 (1703)1720 (1720) 1033 1711 1744 (1744)1762 (1762) 1314 1754 1755 (1763)1781 (1781) 1070 1772 1795 (1795)1813 (1813) 1024 1804 1809 (1809)1832 (1829) 1000 1819 1858 (1860)1882 (1878) 1013 1869 1890 (1890)1914 (1907) 1604 1899 1900 (1904)1930 (1924) 1423 1913 1952 (1952)1971 (1971) 1435 1962 1983 (1983)2003 (2003) 1435 1992 2006 (2009)2035 (2026) 1513 2018 2028 (2033)2054 (2049) 1255 2041 2061 (2061)2080 (2078) 1106 2069 2088 (2091)2109 (2109) 1323 2099 2116 (2118)2136 (2136) 1221 2127 2155 (2157)2175 (2173) 1131 2165 2197 (2197)2215 (2213) 1223 2205 2228 (2230)2248 (2248) 1601 2238 2251 (2254)2273 (2273) 1120 2262 2296 (2296)2318 (2314) 1740 2306 2335 (2337)2358 (2355) 1409 2345 2361 (2361)2384 (2377) 1213 2369 2406 (2406)2431 (2424) 1444 2416 2443 (2443)2470 (2463) 745 2453 2481 (2489)2512 (2505) 1320 2497 2535 (2537)2553 (2553) 1760 2545 2583 (42) 32 (22) 40 2593 1438 (71) 61 (47) 71 24 1074 (155) 145 (131) 155 51 1496 (198) 189 (172) 198 135 1140 (228) 218 (208) 226 181 1003 (239) 227 (217) 236 210 942 (269) 260 (245) 269 217 1199 (317) 307 (297) 315 252 1288 (367) 357 (343) 365 297 1302 (424) 412 (400) 420 348 969 (447) 435 (427) 443 403 957 (485) 473 (465) 481 427 948 (503) 486 (472) 494 465 886 (503) 495 (487) 503 478 867 (517) 507 (490) 515 487 867 (549) 541 (531) 549 497 1237 (578) 569 (560) 578 533 858 (620) 609 (596) 618 560 1084 (655) 647 (636) 655 600 1265 (726) 717 (707) 726 638 1346 (762) 749 (738) 758 707 1156 (797) 786 (776) 797 740 1263 (835) 825 (814) 835 776 1090 (846) 837 (826) 846 816 926 (882) 874 (866) 882 829 1037 (911) 897 (886) 905 866 674 (940) 932 (916) 940 889 1037 (967) 958 (947) 967 923 1371 (1008)1000 (990) 1008 950 1593 (1039)1025 (1016) 1033 992 1294 (1101)1092 (1081)

Done

864 (1242)1232 (1218) 1240 1166 1083 (1272)1261 (1250) 1269 1223 470 (1307)1298 (1286) 1307 1250 668 (1341)1333 (1325) 1341 1289 990 (1396)1388 (1380) 1396 1325 771 (1437)1427 (1415) 1435 1380 1021 (1500)1485 (1476) 1494 1417 611 (1544)1534 (1524) 1542 1476 694 (1573)1565 (1556) 1573 1526 1530 (1612)1600 (1591) 1608 1556 1127 (1671)1660 (1648) 1671 1591 1281 (1706)1694 (1683) 1700 1651 839 (1755)1747 (1737) 1755 1683 1092 (1795)1778 (1768) 1786 1739 765 (1824)1816 (1806) 1824 1770 808 (1853)1841 (1832) 1849 1806 525 (1874)1864 (1856) 1874 1832 669 (1908)1900 (1892) 1908 1856 1255 (1925)1917 (1906) 1925 1892 1170 (1967)1959 (1949) 1967 1909 1035 (2029)2015 (2000) 2024 1949 1426 (2046)2036 (2026) 2046 2007 1133 (2069)2061 (2052) 2069 2026 769 (2107)2099 (2087) 2107 2052 1009 (2173)2163 (2153) 2173 2091 1037 (2199)2188 (2179) 2196 2153 1077 (2247)2237 (2227) 2245 2179 1304 (2274)2262 (2254) 2270 2229 1082 (2306)2298 (2290) 2306 2254 1274 (2345)2337 (2326) 2345 2290 1200 (2425)2409 (2398) 2417 2329 1301 (2499)2489 (2476) 2497 2401 1145 (2513)2504 (2496) 2513 2481 954 (2546)2530 (2517) 2538 2496 1382 (2553)2543 (2534) 2551 2520 1355 (2574)2560 (2550) 2568 2534 1179 (2592)2576 (2561) 2584 2550 1127 (2608)2599 (2588) 2608 2566 985 (2640)2631 (2620) 2640 2591 1242 (2677)2664 (2653) 2673 2622 818 (2719)2711 (2701) 2719 2656 955 (21550)30491 (28020) 17746 2703 13368 (0)29486 (0) 0 12340 0 (0) 0 (0) 0 0 0 0 (0) 0 0 0 (0) 0 0 0 (0) 0 0 0 (0) 0 (0) 0 0 0 (0) 0 (0) 0 (0) 0 0 0 (0) 0 (0) 0 0 0 (0) 0 (0) 0 0 28020 (12340)21550 (17746) 13368 30491 0 (0) 0 (0) 0 28462 0 (0) 0 (0) 0 0 0 (0) 0 (0) 0 0 0 0 (0) 0 0 0 (0) 0 (0) 0 0 0 (0) 0 (0) 0 (0) 0 0 0 (0) 0 (0) 0 0 0 (0) 0 0 (30492) 0 (0) 28020 0 17746 (28462)12340 (13368) 50 21550 0 (0) 0 (0) 0 0 0 (0) 0 (0) 0 0 0 (0) 0 (0) 0 (0) 0 0 0 (0) 0 (0) 0 0 0 (0) 0 0 0 (0) 0 (0) 0 0 0 (0) 0 0 0 (21550)30491 (28020) 17746 0 13368 (0)29742 (0) 0 12340 0 (0) 0 (0) 0 0 0 (0) 0 (0) 0 0 0 (0) 0 (0) 0 (0) 0 0 0 (0) 0 (0) 0 0 0 0 (0) 0 (0) 0 0 0 0 0 26994 (0)24948 (0) 0 27914 0 (0) 0 (0) 0 0 0 (0) 0 (0) 0 0 0 (0) 0 (0) 0 0 0 (0) 0 (0) 0 0 0 (0) 0 (0) 0 0 0 (0) 0 (0) 0 0 0 (17) 0 (0) 0 0 0 (18615) 1 (24078) -27572 0 1338 (-391)-10509 (1624) -29146 -11299 11556 (4011)-26155 (-31534) -11088 31983 -29378 (-3123) 807 (-11780) 9066 -22799 -28408 (-17057)3689 (7254) -24364 -7069 -3070 (15841)-5349 (-13472) -146 -16443 6572 (30675)-323 (29338) 11704 29079 25478 (-13131)20687 (28036) 24882 -17319 17680 (-19705)32721 (27806) -676 8843 -22326 (0)18499 (54) 0 -18003 0 (0) 0 (32704) 688 0 (0) 0 (0) 0 0 0 (0) 0 (0) 0 (0) 0 0 0 (-5568) 0 (0) -5552 0 -5536 (-5504)-5536 (-5520) -5488 -5536 -5456 (-5392)-5392 (-5392) -5392 -5472 -5344 (-5296)-5328 (-5312) -5280 -5360 -5248 (-5184)-5232 (-5216) -5152 -5264 -5136 (-5072)-5104 (-5120) -5024 0 -5056 (-14096)12128 (4) 0 -5040 0 (-8192) 0 (0) 0 0 0 (0) 0 (0) 0 0 0 (0) 0 (0) 0 0 0 (0) 0 (0) 0 0 0 (0) 0 (0) 0 0 0 (0) 0 (0) 0 0 0 (0) 0 0 1 (0)-10318 (256) 0 0 -23564 (0)-2784 (-2880) -2960 0 0 (0) 0 (0) 0 0 0 (0) 0 (0) 0 0 0 (0) 0 (0) 0 0 0 (0) 0 (0) 0 0 0 (0) 0 (0) 0 0 0 (0) 0 (0) 0 0 0 (0) 0 0 2561 0 (0) 0 (0) 0 0 0 (0) 0 (0) 0 0 0 (0) 0 (0) 0 0 0 (0) 0 (0) 0 0 0 (0) 0 (0) 0 0 0 (0) 0 (0) 0 0 0 (0) 0 (0) 0 0 0 (0) 0 (0) 0 0 0 (28013)12077 (12148) 29487 0 28749 (11886)11620 (12081) 13366 25970 25701 (0) 0 (0) 0 28020 0 (0) 0 (0) 0 0 0 (0) 0 0 (0) 0 (0) 0 0 0 (0) 0 (0) 0 0 0 (0) 0 (0) 0 0 0 (0) 0 (0) 0 0 0 (0) 0 (0) 0 0 0 (0) 0 (0) 0 0 0 (0) 0 0 0 (0) 0 (0) 0 0 0 (0) 0 (0) 0 0 0 (0) 0 (0) 0 0 0 (0) 0 (0) 0 0 0 (0) 0 (0) 0 0 0 (0) 0 (0) 0 0 0 (0) 0 (0) 0 0 0 (0) 0 (0) 0 0 0 (

Done

TMpred output for leptin - Mozilla Firefox

File   Edit   View   History   Bookmarks   Tools   Help

0) 0 0 0 (0) 0 (0) 0 0 0 (0) 0 (0) 0 0 0 (0) 0 (0) 0 0 0 (0) 0 (0) 0 0 0 (0) 0 (0) 0 0 0 (0) 0 (0) 0 0 0 (0) 0 (0) 0 0 0 (0) 0 (0) 0 0 0 (0) 0 (0) 0 0 0 (0) 0
(0) 0 0 0 (0) 0 (0) 0 2561 0 (0) 0 (0) 0 0 0 (0) 0 (0) 0 0 0 (0) 0 (0) 0 0 0 (0) 0 (0) 0 0 0 (0) 0 (0) 0 0 0 (0) 0 (0) 0 0 0 (0) 0 (0) 0 0 0 (0) 0 (0) 0 0 0 (
0) 0 (0) 0 0 0 (0) 0 (0) 0 0 0 (0) 0 (0) 0 0 0 (28013)12077 (12148) 29487 0 28749 (11886)11620 (12081) 13366 25970 25701 (0) 0 (0) 0
28020 0 (0) 0 (0) 0 0 0 (0) 0 (0) 0 0 0 (0) 0 (0) 0 0 0 (0) 0 (0) 0 0 0 (0) 0 (0) 0 0 0 (0) 0 (0) 0 0 0 (0) 0 (0) 0 0 0 (0) 0 (0) 0 0 0 (0) 0 (0) 0 0 0 (0) 0
(0) 0 0 0 (0) 0 (0) 0 0 0 (0) 0 (0) 0 0 0 (0) 0 (0) 0 0 0 (0) 0 (0) 0 0 0 (0) 0 (0) 0 0 0 (0) 0 (0) 0 0 0 (0) 0 (0) 0 0 0 (0) 0 (0) 0 0 0 (0) 0 (0) 0 0 0 (0)
0 (0) 0 0 0 (0) 0 (0) 0 0 0 (0) 0 (0) 0 0 0 (0) 0 (0) 0 0 0 (0) 0 (0) 0 0 0 (0) 0 (0) 0 0 0 (0) 0 (0) 0 0 0 (0) 0 (0) 0 0 0 (0) 0 (0) 0 0 0 (0) 0 (0) 0 0 0 (
0) 0 (0) 0 0 0 (0) 0 (0) 0 0 0 (0) 0 (0) 0 0 0 (0) 0 (0) 0 0 0 (0) 0 (0) 0 0 0 (0) 0 (0) 0 0 0 (0) 0 (0) 0 0 0 (0) 0 (0) 0 0 0 (0) 0 (0) 0 0 0 (0) 0 (0) 0 0 0
(0) 0 (0) 0 0 0 (0) 0 (0) 0 0 0 (0) 0 (0) 0 0 0 (0) 0 (0) 0 0 0 (0) 0 (0) 0 0 0 (0) 0 (0) 0 0 0 (0) 0 (0) 0 0 0 (0) 0 (0) 0 0 0 (0) 0 (0) 0 0 0 (0) 0 (0) 0 0
0 (0) 0 (0) 0 0 0 (0) 0 (0) 0 0 0 (0) 0 (0) 0 0 0 (0) 0 (0) 0 0 0 (0) 0 (0) 0 0 0 (0) 0 (0) 0 0 0 (0) 0 (0) 0 0 0 (0) 0 (0) 0 0 0 (0) 0 (0) 0 0 0 (0) 0 (0) 0
0 0 (0) 0 (0) 0 0 0 (0) 0 (0) 0 0 0 (0) 0 (0) 0 0 0 (0) 0 (0) 0 0 0 (0) 0 (0) 0 0 0 (0) 0 (0) 0 0 0 (0) 0 (0) 0 0 0 (0) 0 (0) 0 0 0 (0) 0 (0) 0 0 0 (0) 0 (0)
0 0 0 (0) 0 (0) 0 0 0 (0) 0 (0) 0 0 0 (0) 0 (0) 0 0 0 (0) 0 (0) 0 0 0 (0) 0 (0) 0 0 0 (0) 0 (0) 0 0 0 (0) 0 (0) 0 0 0 (0) 0 (0) 0 0 0 (0) 0 (0) 0 0 0 (0) 0 (
0) 0 0 0 (0) 0 (0) 0 0 0 (0) 0 (0) 0 0 0 (0) 0 (0) 0 0 0 (0) 0 (0) 0 0 0 (0) 0 (0) 0 0 0 (0) 0 (0) 0 0 0 (0) 0 (0) 0 0 0 (0) 0 (0) 0 0 0 (0) 0 (0) 0 0 0 (0) 0
(0) 0 0 0 (0) 0 (0) 0 0 0 (0) 0 (0) 0 0 0 (0) 0 (0) 0 0 0 (0) 0 (0) 0 0 0 (0) 0 (0) 0 0 0 (0) 0 (0) 0 0 0 (0) 0 (0) 0 0 0 (0) 0 (0) 0 0 0 (0) 0 (0) 0 0 0 (0)
0 (0) 0 0 0 (0) 0 (0) 0 0 0 (0) 0 (0) 0 0 0 (0) 0 (0) 0 0 0 (0) 0 (0) 0 0 0 (0) 0 (0) 0 0 0 (0) 0 (0) 0 0 0 (0) 0 (0) 0 0 0 (0) 0 (0) 0 0 0 (0) 0 (0) 0 0 0 (
0) 0 (0) 0 0 0 (0) 0 (0) 0 0 8 (0) 0 (0) 0 0 0 (0) 0 (0) 0 0 0 (0) 0 (0) 0 1 0 (0) 0 (50) 0 0 0 (0) 0 (0) 0 0 -5552 (-5536)-5536 (-5536) -5520 -5568
-5488 (-5392)-5472 (-5456) -5392 -5504 -5392 (-5328)-5360 (-5344) -5312 -5392 -5280 (-5232)-5264 (-5248) -5216 -5296 -5152 (-5104) 0 (-5136)
-5120 -5184 -5024 (0)-5040 (-5056) 1 -5072 256 (0) 0 (0) -19948 -10318 -2880 (0) 0 (-2960) 0 -2784 0 (0) 0 (0) 0 0 0 (0) 0 (0) 0 0 0 (0) 0 (0) 0 0 0 (
0) 0 (0) 0 0 0 (0) 0 (0) 0 0 0 (0) 0 (0) 0 0 0 (0) 0 (0) 0 0 0 (0) 0 (0) 0 0 0 (0) 0 (0) 0 0 0 (0) 0 (0) 0 0 0 (0) 0 (0) 0 0 0 (2561) 0 (0) 0 0 0 (0) 0 (0) 0
0 0 (0) 0 (0) 0 0 0 (0) 0 (0) 0 0 0 (0) 0 (0) 0 0 0 (0) 0 (0) 0 0 0 (0) 0 (0) 0 0 0 (0) 0 (0) 0 0 0 (0) 0 (0) 0 0 0 (0) 0 (0) 0 0 0 (0) 0 (0) 0 0 0 (0) 0 (0)
0 0 -10048 (1) 0 (0) 0 0 0 (0) 0 (0) 0 0 17520 (28528)28512 (28512) 28560 17408 0 (0) 0 (0) 0 28592 0 (0) 0 (0) 0 0 0 (0) 0 (0) 0 0 0 (0)-10319 (
256) 0 0 -19196 (0)-2784 (-2928) -2960 0 0 (0) 0 (0) 0 0 0 (0) 0 (0) 0 0 0 (0) 0 (0) 0 0 0 (0) 0 (0) 0 0 0 (0) 0 (0) 0 0 0 (0) 0 (0) 0 0 0 (0) 0 (0) 0 0 0
(0) 0 (0) 0 0 0 (0) 0 (0) 0 0 0 (0) 0 (0) 0 0 0 (0) 0 (0) 0 0 0 (0) 0 (0) 0 0 0 (0) 0 (0) 0 2561 0 (0) 0 (0) 0 0 0 (0) 0 (0) 0 0 0 (0) 0 (0) 0 0 0 (0) 0 (0)
0 0 0 (0) 0 (0) 0 0 8 (0) 0 (0) 0 0 0 (0) 0 (0) 0 0 0 (0) 0 (0) 0 0 0 (0) 0 (0) 0 0 0 (-10318) 0 (2) 256 0 0 (-2784) 0 (-18588) -2880 0
-2960 (0) 0 (0) 0 0 0 (0) 0 (0) 0 0 0 (0) 0 (0) 0 0 0 (0) 0 (0) 0 0 0 (0) 0 (0) 0 0 0 (0) 0 (0) 0 0 0 (0) 0 (0) 0 0 0 (0) 0 (0) 0 0 0 (0) 0 (0) 0 0 0 (0) 0 (
0) 0 0 0 (0) 0 (0) 0 0 0 (0) 0 (0) 0 0 0 (0)2561 (0) 0 0 0 (0) 0 (0) 0 0 0 (0) 0 (0) 0 0 0 (0) 0 (0) 0 0 0 (0) 0 (0) 0 0 0 (0) 0 (0) 0 0 0 (0) 0 (0) 0 0 0 (
0) 0 (0) 0 0 0 (0) 0 (0) 0 0 0 (0) 0 (0) 0 0 0 (0) 0 (0) 0 0 0 (0) 0 (0) 0 0 0 (1) 0 (0) 0 0 0 (-10318) 0 (2) 256 0 0 (-2784) 0 (-17916)
-2880 0 -2960 (0) 0 (0) 0 0 0 (0) 0 (0) 0 0 0 (0) 0 (0) 0 0 0 (0) 0 (0) 0 0 0 (0) 0 (0) 0 0 0 (0) 0 (0) 0 0 0 (0) 0 (0) 0 0 0 (0) 0 (0) 0 0 0 (0) 0 (0) 0 0
0 (0) 0 (0) 0 0 0 (0) 0 (0) 0 0 0 (0) 0 (0) 0 0 0 (0)2561 (0) 0 0 0 (0) 0 (0) 0 0 0 (0) 0 (0) 0 0 0 (0) 0 (0) 0 0 0 (0) 0 (0) 0 0 0 (0) 0 (0) 0 0 0 (0) 0 (
0) 0 0 0 (0) 0 (0) 0 0 0 (0) 0 (0) 0 0 0 (0) 0 (0) 0 0 0 (0) 0 (0) 25 0 0 (24652)-8148 (0) 0 0 0 (0) 0 (-8036) 0 0 0 (0) 0 (0) 0 0 0 (0) 0 (
0) 0 0 0 (0) 0 (0) 0 0 0 (0)25100 (0) 0 0 0 (0) 0 (0) 0 0 0 (0) 0 (0) 0 0 0 (0) 0 (1) 0 0 0 (0) 0 (0) 0 0 0 (0) 0 (0) 0 0 0 (0) 0 (0) 0 1 0 (0) 0 (0) 25 0 0 (
0) 0 (0) 0 0 0 (0) 0 (0) 0 0 0 (0) 0 (0) 0 0 0 (0) 0 (0) 0 0 0 (0) 0 (0) 0 0 0 (0) 0 (0) 0 0 0 (0) 0 (0) 0 0 0 (0) 0 (0) 0 0 0 (0) 0 (0) 0 0 0 (0) 0 (0) 0 0
17220 (21587)18503 (19787) 86 16660 0 (0) 0 (0) 0 0 0 (0) 0 (0) 0 0 0 (0) 0 (0) 0 0 0 (0) 0 (0) 0 0 0 (0) 0 (0) 0 0 0 (0) 0 (0) 0 0 0 (0)
0 (0) 0 0 0 (0) 0 (0) 0 0 0 (0) 0 (0) 0 0 0 (0) 0 (0) 0 0 0 (0) 0 (0) 0 0 0 (0) 0 (0) 0 0 0 (0) 0 (0) 0 0 0 (0) 0 (0) 0 0 0 (0) 0 (0) 0 0 0 (0)3600 (0) 0 0 0
(-8160) 0 (0) 0 4 0 (0)-8160 (0) 0 0 0 (24608) 0 (0) 0 0 0 (0) 120 (0) 0 0 0 (0) 0 (0) 0 24608 0 (0)-8155 (-8160) 0 0 0 (-10000) 0 (0)
Done

TMpred output for leptin - Mozilla Firefox

File   Edit   View   History   Bookmarks   Tools   Help

0 0 0 (-8160) 0 (0) 0 4 0 (0)-8160 (0) 0 0 0 (24608) 0 (0) 0 0 0 (0) 120 (0) 0 0 0 (0) 0 (0) 0 24608 0 (0)-8155 (-8160) 0 0 0 (-10016) 0 (

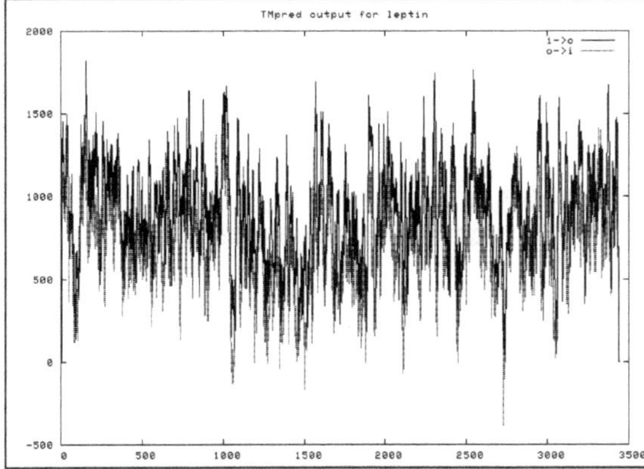

You can get the prediction graphics shown above in one of the following formats:

- GIF-format
- Postscript-format
- numerical format

Back to ISREC home page

Done

TERTIARY STRUCTURE PREDICTION METHOD HOMOLOGY MODELING

Homology Modeling

Homology modeling, also known as **comparative modeling** refers to constructing an atomic-resolution model of the "*target*" protein from its amino acid sequence and an experimental three-dimensional structure of a related homologous protein (the "*template*"). Homology modeling relies on the identification of one or more known protein structures likely to resemble the structure of the query sequence, and on the production of an alignment that maps residues in the query sequence to residues in the template sequence. The sequence alignment and template structure are then used to produce a structural model of the target. Because protein structures are more conserved than DNA sequences, detectable levels of sequence similarity usually imply significant structural similarity.

The quality of the homology model is dependent on the quality of the sequence alignment and template structure. The approach can be complicated by the presence of alignment gaps (commonly called indels) that indicate a structural region present in the target but not in the template, and by structure gaps in the template that arise from poor resolution in the experimental procedure (usually X-ray crystallography) used to solve the structure. Model quality declines with decreasing sequence identity; a typical model has ~1-2 Å root mean square deviation between the matched C^α atoms at 70% sequence identity but only 2-4 Å agreement at 25% sequence identity. However, the errors are significantly higher in the loop regions, where the amino acid sequences of the target and template proteins may be completely different.

Homology modeling can produce high-quality structural models when the target and template are closely related, which has inspired the formation of a structural genomics consortium dedicated to the production of representative experimental structures for all classes of protein folds.

The homology modeling procedure can be broken down into four sequential steps: template selection, target-template alignment, model construction, and model assessment.[1] The first two steps are often essentially performed together, as the most common methods of identifying templates rely on the production of sequence alignments; however, these alignments may not be of sufficient quality because database search techniques prioritize speed over alignment quality. These processes can be performed iteratively to improve the quality of the final model, although quality assessments that are not dependent on the true target structure are still under development.

Aim: To predict the Three Dimensional structure of Ribokinase RBSK(P71913) from MycobacteriumTuberculosis.

Procedure

- Retrieve the protein sequence of Ribokinase from Swissprot database.
- Check the structure availabilty under structure information in Swissprot Entry Form.
- It was observed that there is no PDB structure for the given protein.
- Perform the PDB Blast to know the Sequence similarity towards the Sequence of the Structure in the PDB.
- Observe the Sequence Similarity between the Query and Hits-Select the PDB Structure having Similarity between 25 to 80%.
- Download the PDB Structure which has shown highest similarity between 25 to 80%.
- Open the PDB structure in Swiss PDBviewer using "open"tab in file menu.
- Using load raw sequence in the "Swissmodel" in menu bar
- Fit the raw sequence in the "fit" menu of the menu bar.
- Check the alignment in the window menu.
- Compare the alignment to that of Clustalw and modify the alignment of Swiss PDB using space bar and Del key for inserting gap and deleting the gap.
- Submit the aligned sequence using the submitting swissmodel in the "swissmodel" menu.
- It will generate a PDB document where the swiss PDB is installed.
- Locate the submitted PDB document file to the send request.
- Wait for the mail where it sends the 3D Cordinate files of the target.
- The obtain 3D coordinate file of the target is visualized in Rasmol.
- Check the obtained structure in PROCHECK or with Ramchandranplot in the window menu of Swiss PDB viewer.

Result

3D Structure of the target Ribokinase RBSK was predicted using template of PDB iD 1 RK2A 1and it was checked with swiss PDB Ramchandran plot it has shown following residues in the disallowed regions.

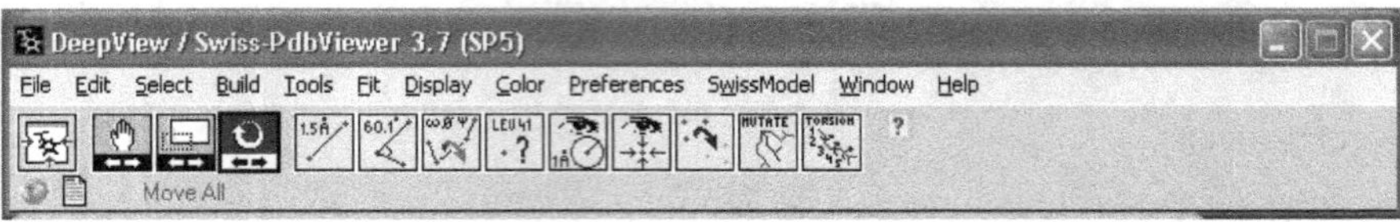

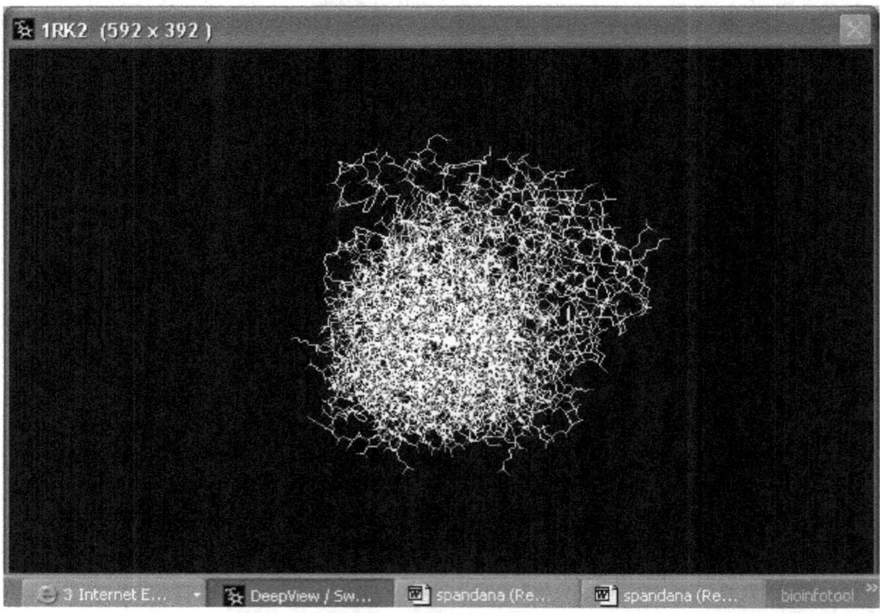

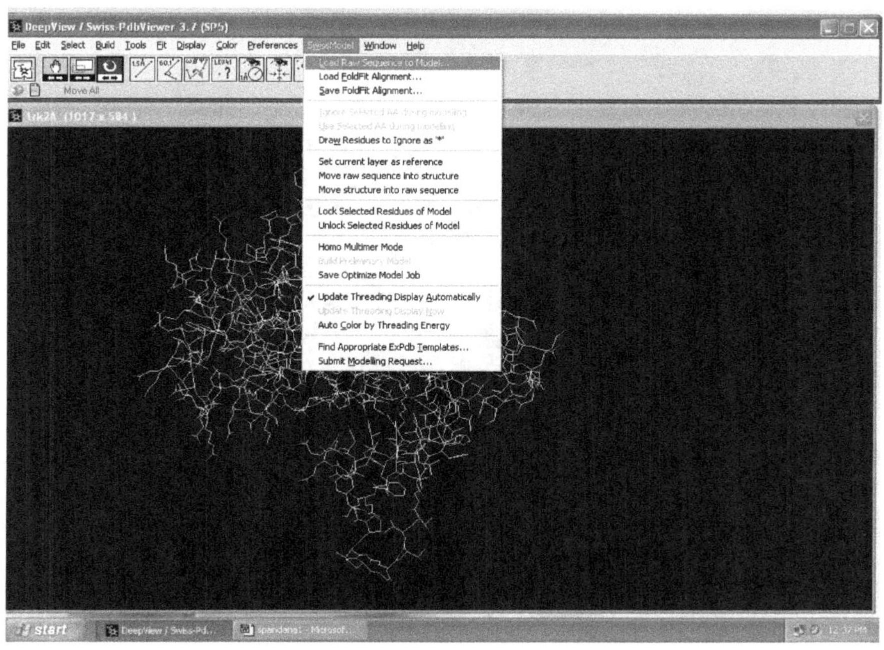

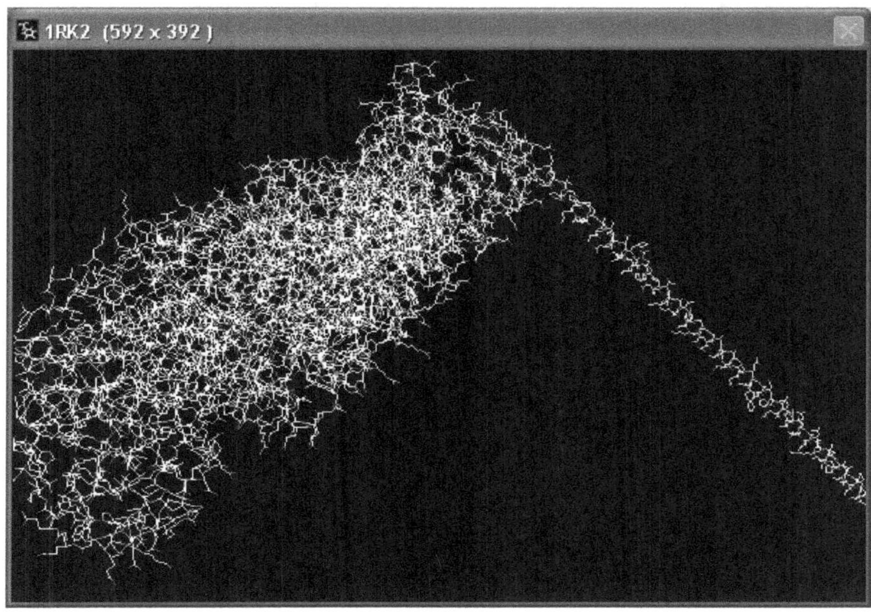

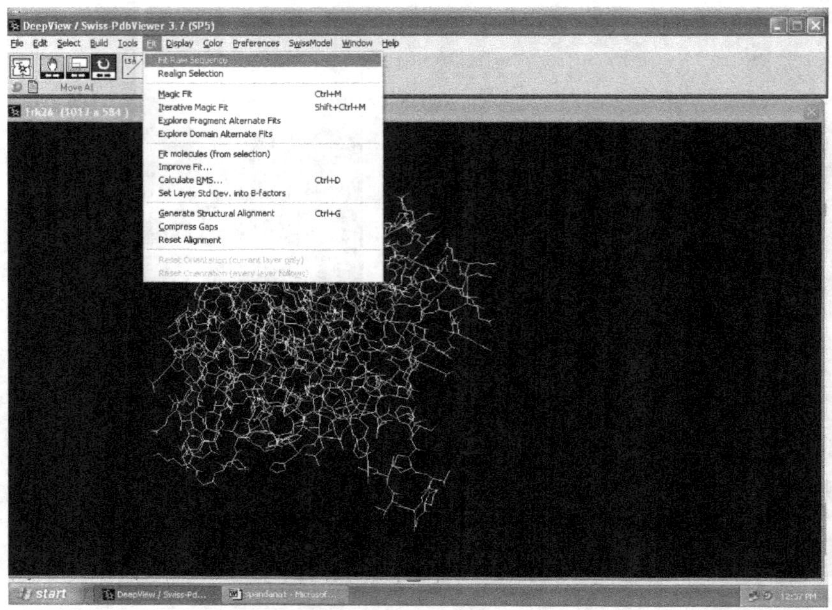

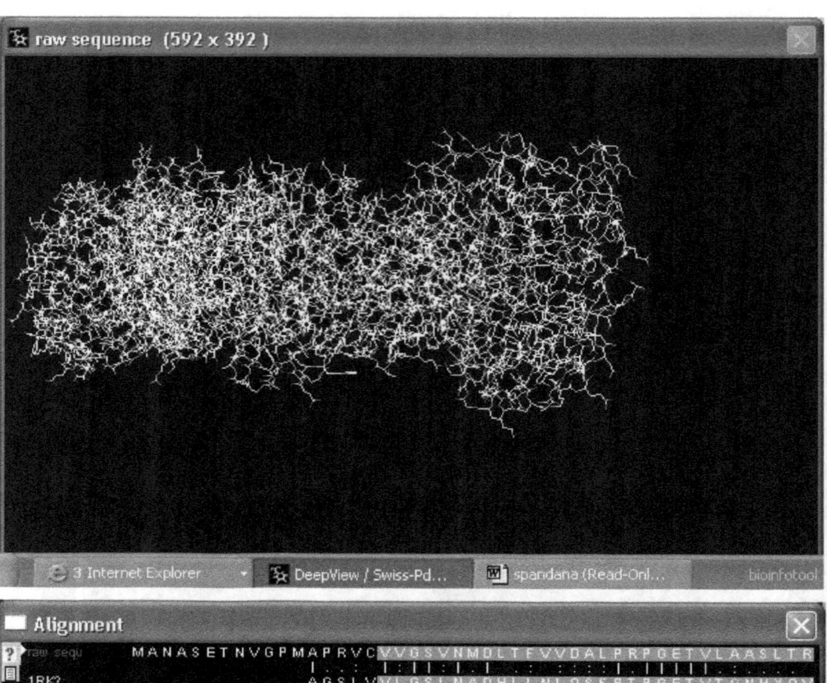

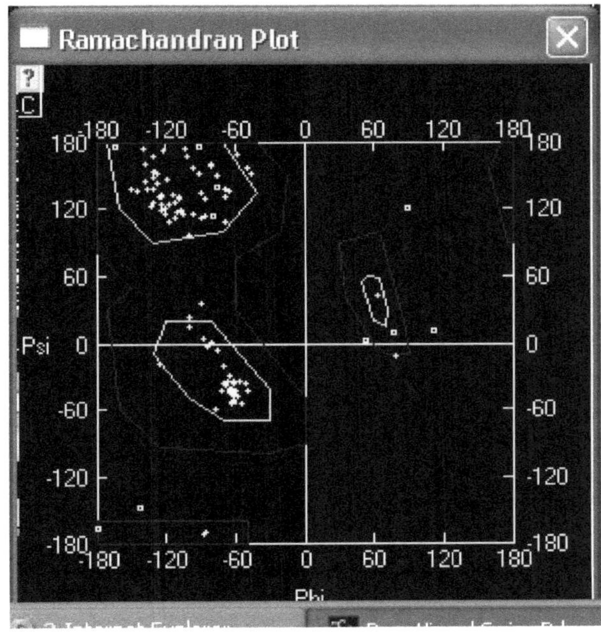

Ramachandran Plot
180   -120   -60   0   60   120   180
180
120
60
Psi   0
-60
-120
-180
-180   -120   -60   0   60   120   180
Phi

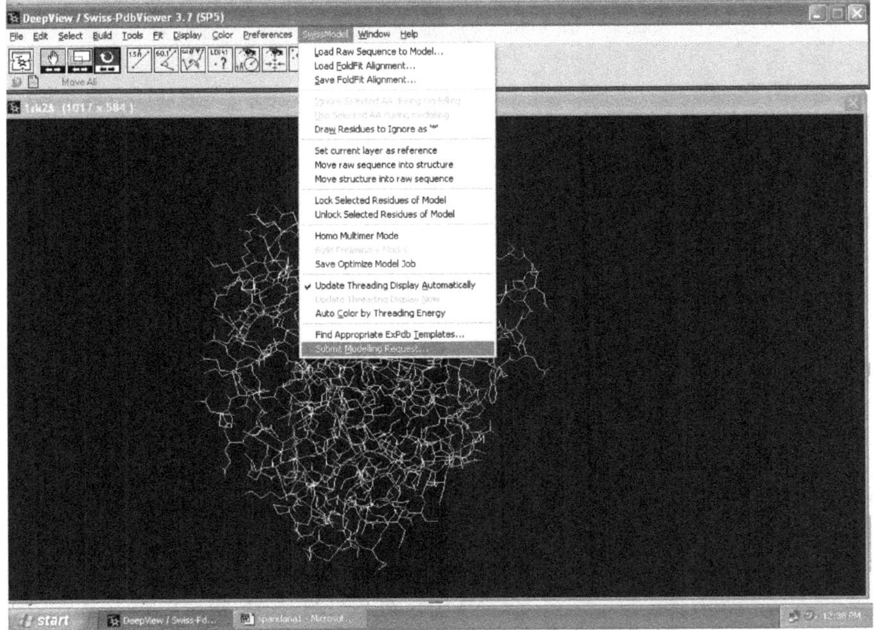

DeepView / Swiss-PdbViewer 3.7 (SP5)
File   Edit   Select   Build   Tools   Fit   Display   Color   Preferences   SwissModel   Window   Help
Move All
1rk2a (1017 x 584)
Load Raw Sequence to Model...
Load FoldFit Alignment...
Save FoldFit Alignment...
Ignore Selected AA during modeling
Use Selected AA during modeling
Draw Residues to Ignore as *
Set current layer as reference
Move raw sequence into structure
Move structure into raw sequence
Lock Selected Residues of Model
Unlock Selected Residues of Model
Homo Multimer Mode
Save Optimize Model Job
Update Threading Display Automatically
Update Threading Display Now
Auto Color by Threading Energy
Find Appropriate ExPdb Templates...
Submit Modeling Request...
start   DeepView / Swiss-Pd...   spandana1 - Microsof...   12:36 PM

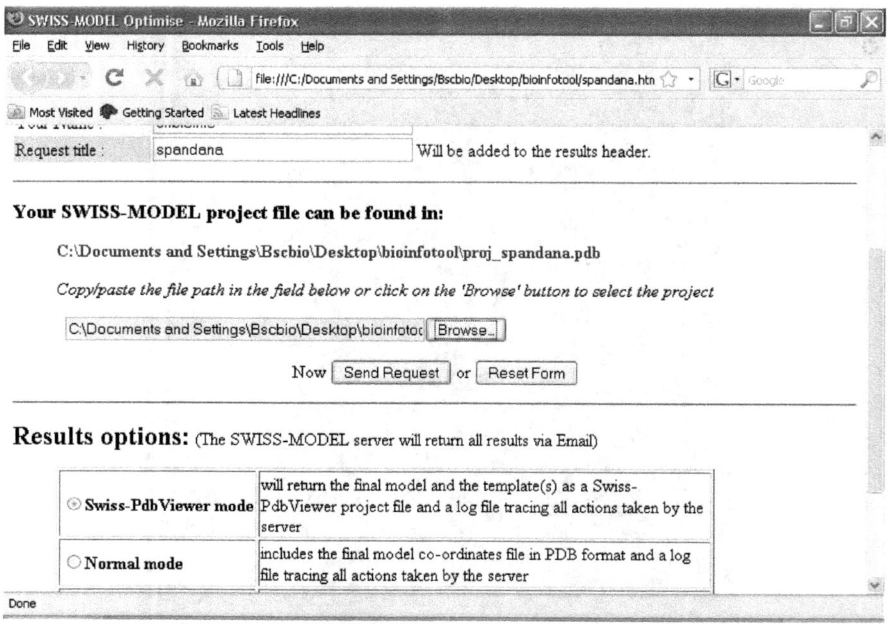

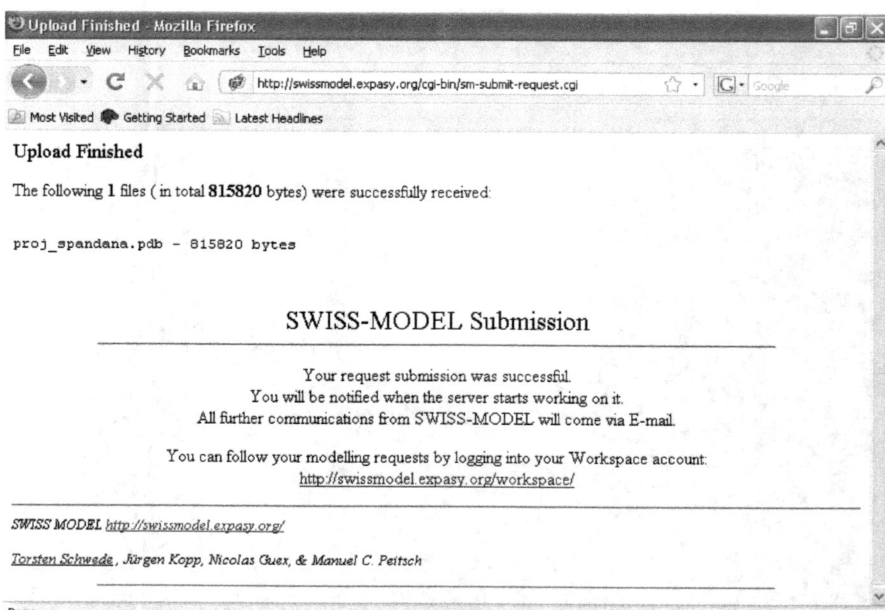

5

STRUCTURE VIZUALISATION TOOLS

RASMOL

RasMol is a molecular graphics program intended for the visualization of proteins, nucleic acids and small molecules.

RasMol has been developed at University of Edinburgh's Biocomputing Research unit and the Bimolecular structure Department, Glaxo Research and Development, Greenford U.K

The program is aimed at display, teaching and generation of publication quality images. RasMol runs on wide range of architectures and operating systems including Microsoft Windows, Apple Macintosh, UNIX and VMS systems. UNIX and VMS versions have some exceptions. For details, search installation page at RasMol server.

The program reads in a molecule coordinate file and interactively displays the molecule on the screen in a variety of color schemes and molecule representations. Currently available representations include depth-cued wireframes, 'Dreiding' sticks, space filling (CPK) spheres, ball and stick, solid and strand bimolecular ribbons, atom labels and dot surfaces.

Up to 5 molecules may be loaded and displayed at once. Any one or all of the molecules may be rotated and translated.

The program reads in molecular coordinate files and interactively displays the molecule on the screen in a variety of representations and color schemes. Supported input file formats include Protein Data Bank (PDB), Tripos Associates' Alchemy and Sybyl Mol2 formats, Molecular Design Limited's (MDL) Mol file format, Minnesota Supercomputer Center's (MSC) XYZ (XMol) format, CHARMm format, CIF format and mmCIF format files. If connectivity information is not contained in the file this is calculated automatically.

The loaded molecule can be shown as wireframe bonds, cylinder 'Dreiding' stick bonds, alpha-carbon trace, space-filling (CPK) spheres, macromolecular ribbons (either smooth shaded solid ribbons or parallel strands), hydrogen bonding and dot surface representations. Atoms may also be labeled with arbitrary text strings. Alternate conformers and multiple NMR models may be specially colored and identified in atom labels. Different parts of the molecule may be represented and colored independently of the rest of the molecule or displayed in several representations simultaneously.

The displayed molecule may be rotated, translated, zoomed and z-clipped (slabbed) interactively using either the mouse, the scroll bars, the command line or an attached dial box. RasMol can read a prepared list of commands from a 'script' file (or via inter-process communication) to allow a given image or viewpoint to be restored quickly. RasMol can also create a script file containing the commands required to regenerate the current image. Finally, the rendered image may be written out in a variety of formats including either raster or vector PostScript, GIF, PPM, BMP, PICT, Sun raster file or as a MolScript input script or Kinemage.

Command References

RasMol allows the execution of interactive commands typed at the **'RasMol>'** prompt in the terminal window. Each command must be given on a separate line. Keywords are case insensitive and may be entered in either upper or lower case letters. All whitespace characters are ignored except to separate keywords and their arguments.

The commands/keywords currently recognised by RasMol are given below.

Backbone

Syntax: backbone {<boolean>}
        backbone <value>
        backbone dash

Background

Syntax: background <colour>

Cartoon

Syntax: cartoon {<number>}

Ribbons

Syntax: ribbons {<boolean>}
        ribbons <value>

Colour

Syntax: colour {<object>} <colour>
        color {<object>} <colour>

HBonds

Syntax: hbonds {<boolean>}

    hbonds <value>

Select

Syntax: select {<expression>}

Script

Syntax: script <filename>

Set

Syntax: set <parameter> {<option>}

Show

Syntax: show information

    show centre

    show phipsi

    show RamPrint

    show rotation

    show selected { group | chain | atom }

    show sequence

    show symmetry

    show translation

    show zoom

Spacefill

Syntax: spacefill {<boolean>}

    spacefill temperature

    spacefill user

    spacefill <value>

SSBonds

Syntax: ssbonds {<boolean>}

    ssbonds <value>

Structure

Syntax: structure

Label

Syntax: label {<string>}

    label <boolean>

The following table lists the current expansion specifiers:

%a	Atom Name
%b %t	B-factor/Temperature
%c %s	Chain Identifier
%e	Element Atomic Symbol
%i	Atom Serial Number
%n	Residue Name
%r	Residue Number
%M	NMR Model Number (with leading "/")
%A	Alternate Conformation Identifier (with leading ";")

Show

Syntax: show information

    show centre

    show phipsi

    show RamPrint

    show rotation

    show selected { group | chain | atom }

    show sequence

    show symmetry

    show translation

    show zoom

Zoom

Syntax: zoom {<boolean>}

    zoom <value>

Set Hetero

Syntax: set hetero <boolean>

Within Expressions

select within(3.2,backbone)'

Translate

Syntax: translate <axis> {-} <value>

Save

Syntax: save {pdb} <filename>

   save mdl <filename>

   save alchemy <filename>

   save xyz <filename>

Rotate

Syntax: rotate <axis> {-} <value>

   rotate bond {<boolean>}

   rotate molecule {<boolean>}

   rotate all {<boolean>}

Aim: To find the Ligand Active site of Human Alcohol Dehydrogenase (AccNo.......). 2W98

Procedure

- Retrieve Alcohol Dehydrogenase of [2W98] from Protein Data Bank(PDB) and Download the Pdb file at the Desktop.
- Initiate Rasmol at the Desktop.
- With the help of "Open" tab in the File Menu of Rasmol Tool, Browse the Downloaded Pdb File. (Rasmol permits representation of polypeptide in Ball&Stick Model)
- (Type "Select all" command on command line prompt to select all the atoms of residues of a protein.)
- "Select Hetero" on command line, selects the Hetero atom of the given Pdb file
- The currently selected atoms are represented in the solid sphere by "Spacefill True" on command line prompt.
- To demark the selected Hetero Atom in Red color using Color command [Color Red].
- By using "Within Expression" command the Hetero atoms interacting with the proximal Aminoacids of the given protein is performed [Select within (4.0, Hetero)].
- With Label command the Aminoacids interacting with the heteroatoms are labeled.
- The Hydrogen bonding Label between the interacting residues to the hetero atom was observed using "HydrogenBond" on Syntax.

- The labelled residues are known to be a part of the Hetero Atom active site.

Results: The following residues may play a vital role in Hetero Atom active site of the given protein.

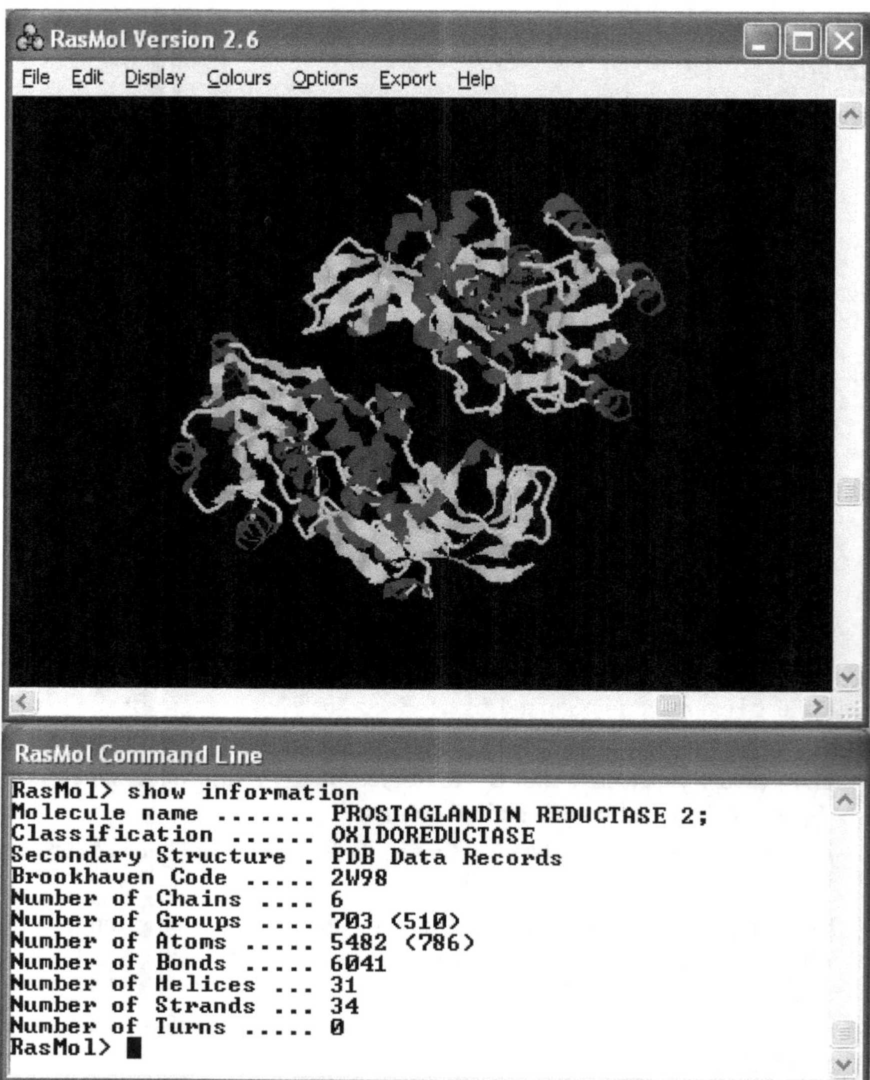

6

MOLECULAR MODELLING

Cn3D

Cn3D is a Windows, Macintosh and Unix-based software from the <u>United States National Library of Medicine</u> that acts as a helper application for web browsers to view three-dimensional structures from The <u>National Center for Biotechnology Information</u>'s <u>Entrez</u> retrieval service. It "simultaneously displays structure, sequence, and alignment, and now has powerful annotation and alignment editing features".

Cn3D is a visualization tool for bimolecular structures, sequences, and sequence alignments. What sets Cn3D apart from other software is its ability to correlate structure and sequence information: for example, a scientist can quickly find the residues in a crystal structure that correspond to known disease mutations, or conserved active site residues from a family of sequence homologs. Cn3D displays structure-structure alignments along with their structure-based sequence alignments, to emphasize what regions of a group of related proteins are most conserved in structure and sequence. Also included are custom labeling features, high-quality <u>OpenGL</u> graphics, and a variety of file exports that together make Cn3D a powerful tool for literature annotation. Cn3D is typically run from a WWW browser as a helper application for NCBI's <u>Entrez</u> system, but it can also be used as a standalone application.

Cn3D intentionally does not read PDB-format files directly, but instead uses NCBI's <u>MMDB database</u>. Briefly, MMDB takes data from the <u>Protein Data Bank</u>, parses each PDB file in order to perform extensive validation and error correction, and stores the information in a more computer-friendly format.

Aim: To visualize the 3D structure of PTEN tumor suppressor protein (1D5R) using Cn3D.

Procedure

- Retrieve the MMDB format files of 1D5R from Molecular Modelling DataBase of NCBI.

- Invoke Cn3D on the Desktop, using file menu open the 1D5R MMDB file.
- It depicts the structure colorfully and interactively.
- The whole structure can be made larger or smaller with **View:Zoom In** and **View:Zoom Out**.
- The view returned to its original size and orientation as stored in the data file with **View:Restore**. **View:Reset** will fit the entire structure into the window.

Result: The 1D5R structure was visualized interactively.

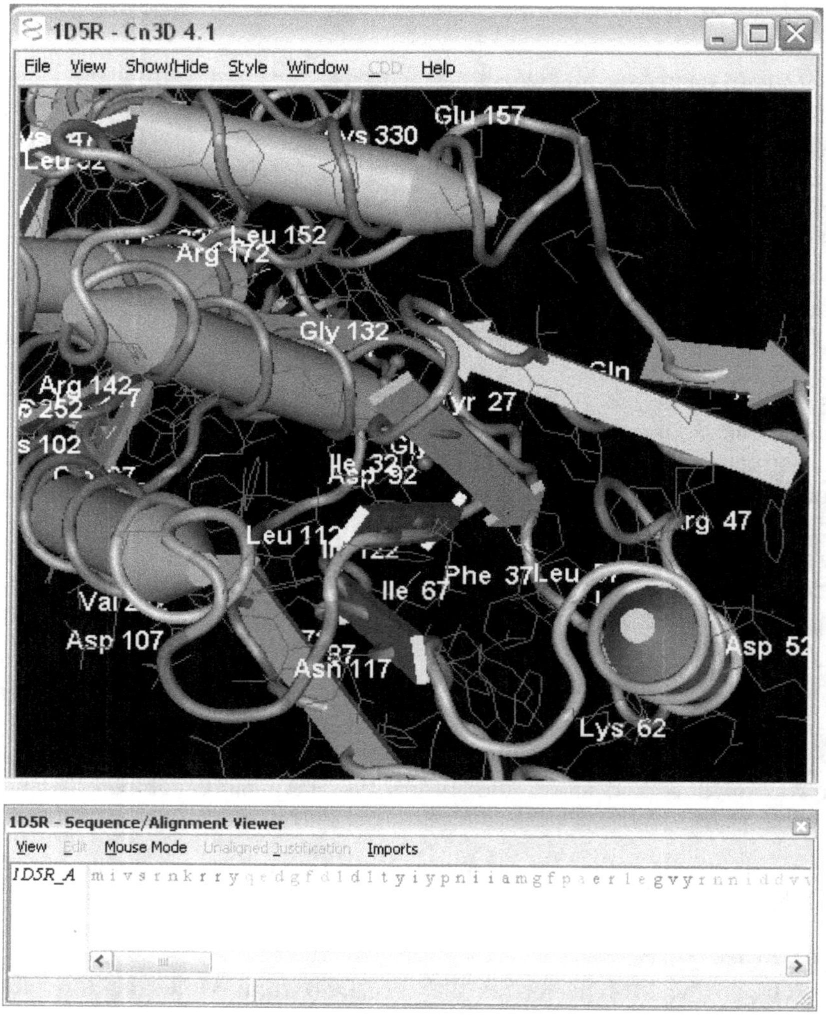

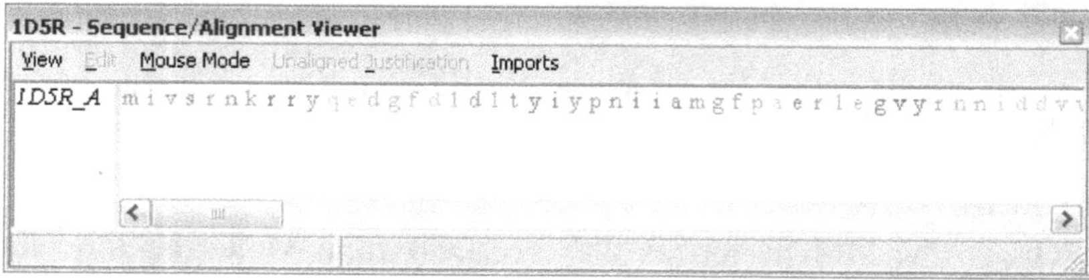

Drug Designing

Drug design also sometimes referred to as **rational drug design** is the inventive process of finding new medications based on the knowledge of the biological target. The drug is most commonly a organic small molecule which activates or inhibits the function of a biomolecule such as a protein which in turn results in a therapeutic benefit to the patient. In the most basic sense, drug design involves design of small molecules that are complementary in shape and charge to the biomolecular target to which they interact and therefore will bind to it. Drug design frequently but not necessarily relies on computer modeling techniques. This type of modeling often referred to as **computer-aided drug design**.

Typically a drug target is a key molecule involved in a particular metabolic or signaling pathway that is specific to a disease condition or pathology, or to the infectivity or survival of a microbial pathogen. Some approaches attempt to inhibit the functioning of the pathway in the diseased state by causing a key molecule to stop functioning. Drugs may be designed that bind to the active region and inhibit this key molecule. Another approach may be to enhance the normal pathway by promoting specific molecules in the normal pathways that may have been affected in the diseased state. In addition, these drugs should also be designed in such a way as not to affect any other important "off-target" molecules that may be similar in appearance to the target molecule since drug interactions with off-target molecules may lead to undesirable side effects. Sequence homology is often used to identify such risks.

One can design a molecular compound based on the active site of the protein using softwares like ISIS/Draw, Chemdraw , chemsketch , Arguslab and many QSAR softwares.

The current book further aims for description of the how to Develop 3D-co ordinates of the any drug molecule to visualize and analyze the structure in either visualization tools or for Drug-Target docking studies.

ArgusLab : Planaria Software freely distributes its molecular modeling and drug-design program, ArgusLab to anyone who desires a license. It is used world-wide in teaching and industry for teaching, spectroscopy, graphics & visualization, drug-docking, and high-level ab initio calculations. It is available at http://www.arguslab.com

CHEMSKETCH

This is an introduction to the program ChemSketch, from ACD Labs. You can use ChemSketch to draw chemical structures, and to view them as three dimensional (3D) models.

Aim: To draw the propane structure using ChemSketch.

Procedure

- Invoke the shortcut of chemsketch tool on the desktop.
- Two of the tool buttons are litted up when ChemSketch is invoked(1.Structure-upper row of buttons, at left 2.In left side of buttons 'c')
- Single click any where on the main screen displays CH_4.
- Twice click on the position of the 'C' atom on CH_4, completes the propane structure.
- The drawn structure is 3D optimized and save the file mol format.
- Visualize the 3D structure using Rasmol.

Result

The propane 2D structure was drawn and 3D structure was viewed in Rasmol.

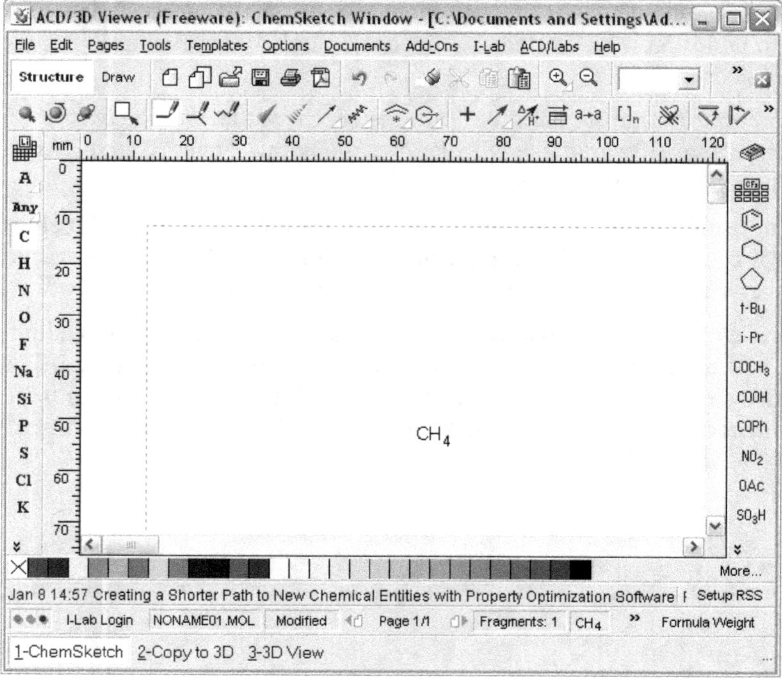

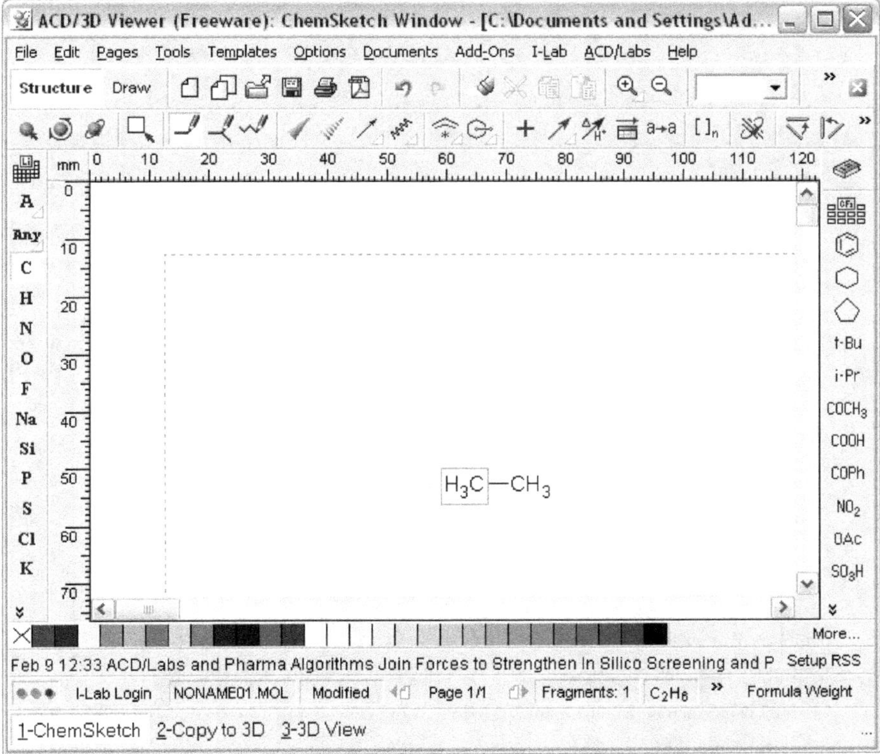

ACD/3D Viewer (Freeware): ChemSketch Window - [C:\Documents and Settings\Ad...
File   Edit   Pages   Tools   Templates   Options   Documents   Add-Ons   I-Lab   ACD/Labs   Help
Structure   Draw
H₃C—CH₃
t-Bu
i-Pr
COCH₃
COOH
COPh
NO₂
OAc
SO₃H
More...
Feb 9 12:33 ACD/Labs and Pharma Algorithms Join Forces to Strengthen In Silico Screening and P   Setup RSS
I-Lab Login   NONAME01.MOL   Modified   Page 1/1   Fragments: 1   C₂H₆   Formula Weight
1-ChemSketch   2-Copy to 3D   3-3D View

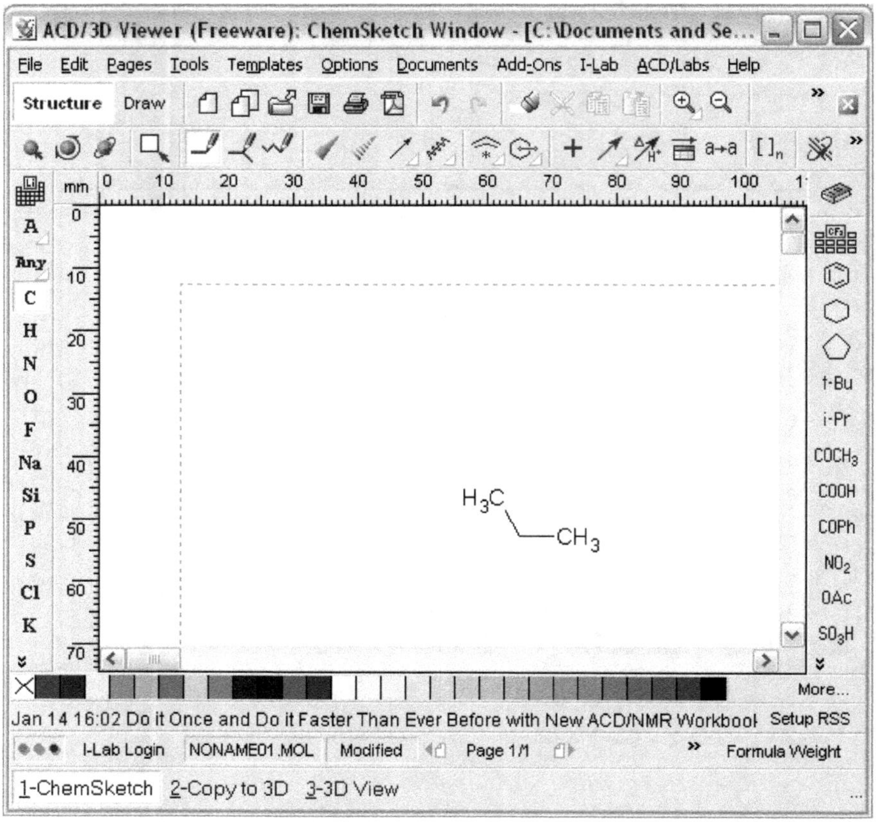

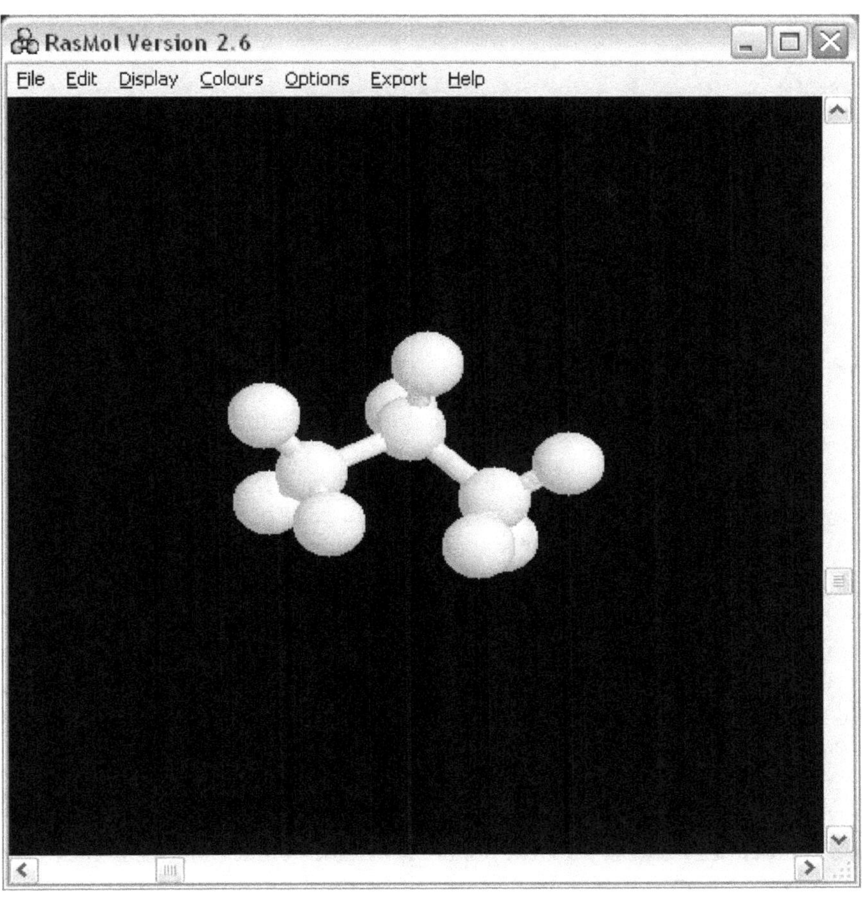

RasMol Version 2.6
File   Edit   Display   Colours   Options   Export   Help

7

DRUG – DOCKING

DOCKING

In the field of <u>molecular modeling</u>, **docking** is a method which predicts the preferred orientation of one molecule to a second when <u>bound</u> to each other to form a stable <u>complex</u>.[1] Knowledge of the preferred orientation in turn may be used to predict the strength of association or <u>binding affinity</u> between two molecules using for example <u>scoring functions</u>.

The associations between biologically relevant molecules such as <u>proteins</u>, <u>nucleic acids</u>, <u>carbohydrates</u>, and <u>lipids</u> play a central role in <u>signal transduction</u>. Furthermore, the relative orientation of the two interacting partners may affect the type of signal produced (e.g., <u>agonism</u> vs <u>antagonism</u>). Therefore docking is useful for predicting both the strength and type of signal produced.

Docking is frequently used to predict the binding orientation of <u>small molecule</u> <u>drug</u> candidates to their protein targets in order to, in turn, predict the affinity and activity of the small molecule. Hence docking plays an important role in the <u>rational design of drugs</u>.[2] Given the biological and <u>pharmaceutical</u> significance of molecular docking, considerable efforts have been directed towards improving the methods used to predict docking .

Applications

A binding interaction between a small molecule ligand and an <u>enzyme</u> protein may result in activation or <u>inhibition</u> of the enzyme. If the protein is a receptor, ligand binding may result in <u>agonism</u> or <u>antagonism</u>. Docking is most commonly used in the field of <u>drug design</u> — most drugs are small <u>organic</u> molecules, and docking may be applied to:

> ➢ Hit identification – docking combined with a <u>scoring function</u> can be used to quickly screen large databases of potential drugs <u>in silico</u> to identify molecules that are likely to bind to protein target of interest (see <u>virtual screening</u>).

➢ Lead optimization – docking can be used to predict in where and in which relative orientation a ligand binds to a protein (also referred to as the binding mode or pose). This information may in turn be used to design more potent and selective analogs.

➢ Bioremediation – Protein ligand docking can also be used to predict pollutants that can be degraded by enzymes.[1]

Aim: To Dock the inhibitor benzamidine into to the serine protease beta trypsin.

Procedure

- Retrieve the PDB format files of ligand and protein.
- Load the protein and ligand in arguslab.
- Select the ligand alone and hide the remaining molecules.
- Add hydrogens to the ligand molecule using shift and H button on the tool bar.
- Make a replica of ligand by using ctrl+c and ctrl+v.
- Repeat the step 4 for the new Benzamidine.
- Under groups folder of residue in the tree view one can observe two ligands i.e 1BEN and 2BEN.
- Modify the names 1BEN – Ligand_xray and 2BEN- Ligand by right click on the molecules and using "Modify group's" option.
- Make the binding site for the ligand-xray group. The easy way is to right-click on the ligand-xray group in the Groups folder and select the "Make a BindingSite Group for this Group" menu option
- Bring up the Dock Settings dialog box by selecting the Calculation/Dock a Ligand... menu option or clicking on the "H" button on the toolbar.
- Select the ligand to dock in the "Ligand" drop-box. Make sure to select the group named "ligand" group and NOT the "ligand-xray" group.
- Click on the "Calculate Size" button and a docking box tailored to the binding site will be make and shown on the screen. Make sure "ArgusDock" is the docking engine, the Calculation type = Dock, and the Ligand is Flexible.
- Click the "Start" button and the docking calculation will begin.

Result

Inhibitor benzamidine got docked into to the serine protease beta trypsin, Pose 2 of the given docking results shown to be best pose with minimum energy.

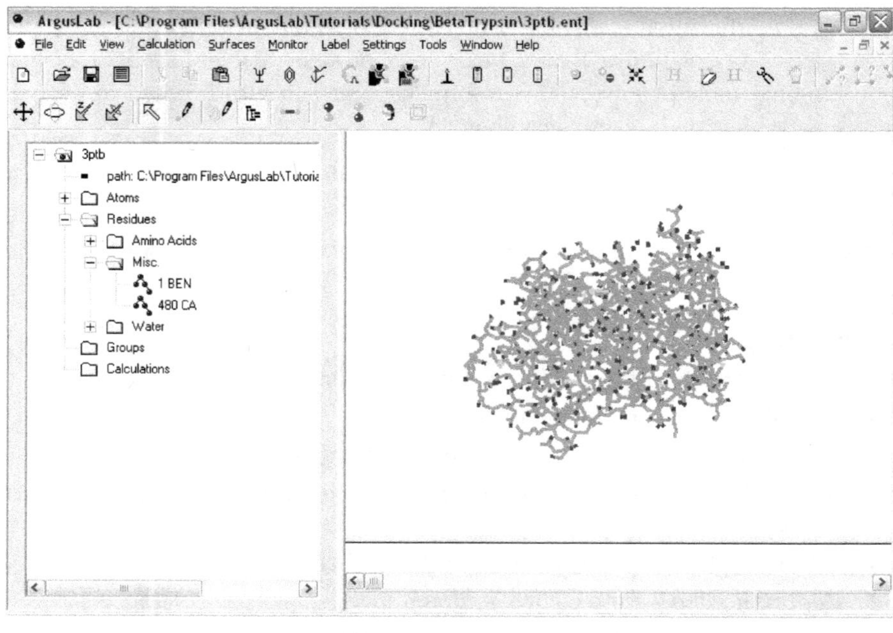

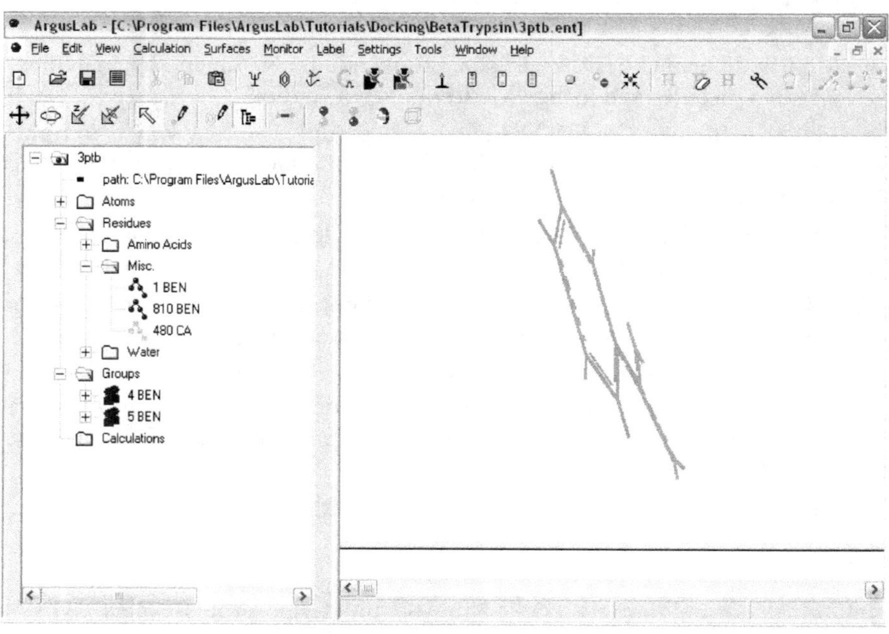

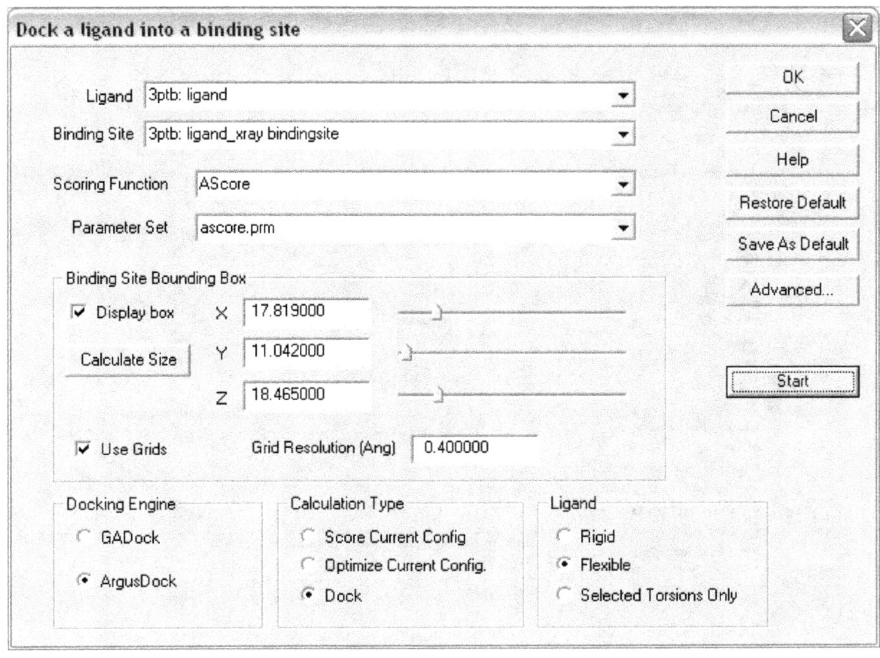

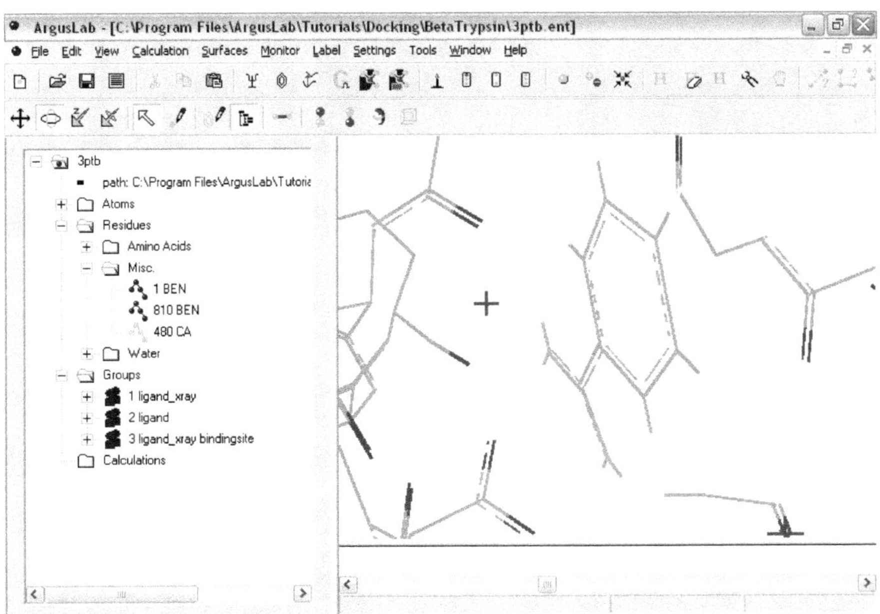

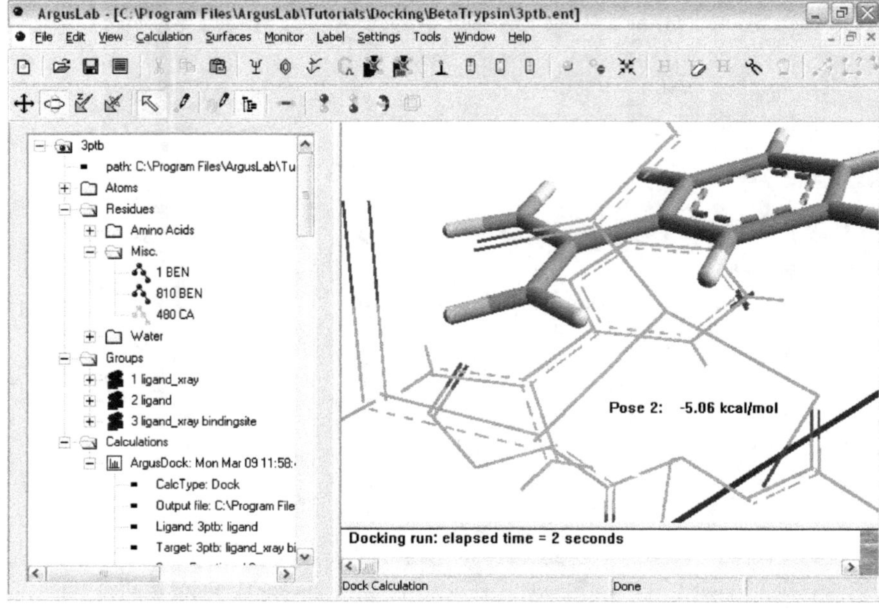

ArgusLab - [C:\Program Files\ArgusLab\Tutorials\Docking\BetaTrypsin\3ptb.ent]
File   Edit   View   Calculation   Surfaces   Monitor   Label   Settings   Tools   Window   Help
3ptb
path: C:\Program Files\ArgusLab\Tu
Atoms
Residues
Amino Acids
Misc.
1 BEN
810 BEN
480 CA
Water
Groups
1 ligand_xray
2 ligand
3 ligand_xray bindingsite
Calculations
ArgusDock: Mon Mar 09 11:58:
CalcType: Dock
Output file: C:\Program File
Ligand: 3ptb: ligand
Target: 3ptb: ligand_xray bi
Pose 2:   -5.06 kcal/mol
Docking run: elapsed time = 2 seconds
Dock Calculation
Done